# MENTAL HEALTH CARE FOR ALLIED HEALTH AND NURSING PROFESSIONALS

# DEDICATION

*To our families, who are our emotional support,*
*and*
*To all the health care workers,*
*who will help take care*
*of the mental health of our patients*

# MENTAL HEALTH CARE FOR ALLIED HEALTH AND NURSING PROFESSIONALS

*Edited by*

## H. STEVEN MOFFIC, M.D.
## PEDRO RUIZ, M.D.
## GEORGE L. ADAMS, M.D.

*Department of Psychiatry*
*Baylor College of Medicine*
*Houston, Texas*

*With 21 Contributors*

**WARREN H. GREEN, INC.**
St. Louis, MO, U.S.A.

*Published by*

**WARREN H. GREEN, INC.**
8356 Olive Boulevard
St. Louis, Missouri 63132, U.S.A.





*ISBN No. 0-87527-344-0*

# LIST OF CONTRIBUTING AUTHORS

GEORGE L. ADAMS, M.D.
Professor of Psychiatry, Dartmouth
Hanover, N.H.

TIMOTHY L. BAYER, M.D.
Assistant Professor of Psychiatry
Baylor College of Medicine
Houston, Texas

JOAN BROCHSTEIN, M.S.W., M.P.H.
Private Practice of Social Work
Houston, Texas

RICHARD CARLSON, M.D.
Assistant Professor of Psychiatry
Baylor College of Medicine
Houston, Texas

RANJIT C. CHACKO, M.D.
Assistant Professor of Psychiatry
Baylor College of Medicine
Houston, Texas

LOIS C. FRIEDMAN, Ph.D.
Assistant Professor of Psychology
Baylor College of Medicine
Houston, Texas

EFRAIN A. GOMEZ, M.D.
Department of Psychiatry
Veterans Administration Hospital
Houston, Texas

BEVERLY HERBERT, B.S., R.N.
Office of Public Affairs
Baylor College of Medicine
Houston, Texas

DARYL K. KNOX, M.D.
Assistant Professor of Psychiatry
Baylor College of Medicine
Houston, Texas

RAMON A. LAVAL, Ph.D.
Assistant Professor of Psychology
Baylor College of Medicine
Houston, Texas

BRUCE MARSH, Ph.D.
Assistant Professor of Psychology
Baylor College of Medicine
Houston, Texas

H. STEVEN MOFFIC, M.D.
Associate Professor of Psychiatry
Baylor College of Medicine
Houston, Texas

GUY K. PATTERSON, M.D.
Private Practice of Psychiatry
Houston, Texas

OCTAVIO C. PINELL, M.D.
Associate Professor of Psychiatry
Baylor College of Medicine
Houston, Texas

JESSE REED, Ph.D.
Assistant Professor of Psychology
Baylor College of Medicine
Houston, Texas

LAWRENCE ROOT, M.D.
Private Practice of Psychiatry
Houston, Texas

PEDRO RUIZ, M.D.
Professor and Vice-Chairman
Department of Psychiatry
Baylor College of Medicine
Houston, Texas

PEDRO P. RUIZ
Pre-Medicine Undergraduate Student
Houston, Texas

PONCE SANDLIN, M.D.
Department of Psychiatry
Veterans Administration Hospital
Houston, Texas

EDWARD G. SILVERMAN, Ph.D.
Assistant Professor of Psychology
Byalor College of Medicine
Houston, Texas

SETH W. SILVERMAN, M.D.
Private Practice of Psychiatry
Houston, Texas

# ACKNOWLEDGMENTS

The editors would like to express particular appreciation to Robert L. Williams, M.D. and Alex D. Pokorny, M.D., whose leadership inspired those of us who worked on this book. In addition, the completion of the manuscript was aided by the expert secretarial assistance of Barbara DuMensil and Hady Sanchez.

# CONTENTS

# MENTAL HEALTH CARE FOR ALLIED HEALTH AND NURSING PROFESSIONALS

# Chapter 1

SOME BASIC FACTS ABOUT MENTAL DISORDERS

GUY K. PATTERSON, M.D.

In spite of an impressive literature on mental disorders, these conditions are draped in ambivalent images and metaphors. On the one hand, individuals with mental disorders are dangerous; they are the psychotic killers talking on the screens of television and the cinema. On the other hand, they are fragile, delicate victims of society driven crazy by institutions and indifference. This imagery is to be expected because any important condition, whose causality is murky and whose treatment is often ineffective, takes on extra meaning.

Metaphors and myths about mental disorders prevail. Few people know the symptoms of mental disorders; they often equate mental disorders with violent behavior. Many have misconceptions about the causes of mental disorders, accepting the notion that "people can crack under stress" but dismissing the fact that disorders can run in families and can be caused by disorders in the central nervous system. Some feel that mental illness is the result of moral failing or lack of will power. Single causes or explanations are often sought. Treatment is also misunderstood. Medications for mental disorders are felt to be crutches; psychotherapy, pablum for the wealthy. Psychiatric hospitals are places to be avoided unless the patient is dangerous. State hospitals are still felt to be snake pits. Patients with mental illness are stigmatized; people are frightened and repelled by them. The patients themselves have misconceptions which alter their self-image and self-esteem.

You, as perspective caregivers, must examine your notions and fears about mental disorders because they will ultimately affect the quality of your care. Many of your patients will have both mental disorders and medical diseases. In 1978, a presidential commission on mental health showed that seven million poeple, or three percent of the U.S. population, were seen hospitalized in mental hospitals. The commission estimated that at any one time about 15 percent of U.S. citizens need some form of mental health service (1).

## DEFINING MENTAL ILLNESS

The third edition of The Diagnostic and Statistical Manual of Mental Disorders of the American Psychiatric Association, better known as DSM III, defines and classifies mental disorders. The manual which took five years to develop, involving many field trials with clinicians, brings diagnostic stability and consistency to American psychiatry. According to DSM III, mental disorders "are clinically significant behavioral or psychological syndromes or patterns that occur in an individual and that are typically associated with either a painful symptom (distressed) or impairment in one or more important areas of functioning (disability)."

Mental disorders share several important characteristics. People don't just have nervous breakdowns or become disturbed. They experience specific symptoms at certain times and their symptoms follow a course. For example, a person with schizophrenia in order to be considered schizophrenic must have specific symptoms at specific times. That person must have auditory hallucinations, delusions, and incoherence for at least six months. There must be some deterioration in social functioning at work or at home. There must also be historical evidence from the family or presence of other symptoms like withdrawal or social isolation. Schizophrenia, like multiple sclerosis or diabetes, is not inevitably progressive. There are times when a person with schizophrenia is in remission and in fact is not behaving or appearing schizophrenically at all (2).

## DIAGNOSING MENTAL DISORDERS

Perceptive students will notice that DSM III refers to mental disorders rather than diseases. This distinction is important for a number of reasons. Disorders are deviations from what is normal or what is expected. Diseases are also deviations from normal states of health but usually causitive agents and pathological lesions can be identified.

Psychiatry has lagged behind the rest of medicine, certainly not for lack of effort in identifying causes for psychiatric disorders. Most psychiatric diagnosis begins and ends with a careful description of signs and symptoms. Ultimate confirming causes for these disorders can rarely be identified.

More than other medial specialities, psychiatric diagnosis relies upon nosology. Nosology is the science of the classification of diseases. The skilled mental health professional must listen carefully for the progression of symptoms. Is the patient anxious? Does he have "nervous attacks," palpitations and sweating? Does he feel afraid? For how long? Does it occur in attacks or is it present all the time? How long has he felt this way? The clinician must also be a skilled observer of behavior. Does the patient look apprehensive? Is he grimacing? Sweating? Hyperventilating? Is he calmly describing the episode?

The patterns of symptoms and the course of the major mental disorders have been defined and redefined more precisely over the past one hundred years, but confusing matters, important medical diseases often mimic mental disorders.


## CAUSES OF MENTAL DISORDERS

Ultimate causes for mental disorders are not known; they are usually multi-determined like cancer, heart disease, stroke, and other chronic conditions. Scientists looking for the causes of mental disorders such as psychiatrists, psychologists, neurochemists, psychoanalysts, behaviorists, psychiatric sociologists and many others approach the problem of etiology in many different ways. The analogy of the blind men and the elephant applies both to medical disease and mental disorders, but in the case of mental disorders, the blind men often do not speak the same language and tend to misunderstand each other.

Dialogues about the causes of mental disorders are often heated because there are different traditions of investigation. Biological researchers like neurophysiologists, psychopharmacologists, biological psychiatrists direct their inquiries into the physical, organic world. We see their results in the exciting discoveries of the anti-psychotic and anti-depressant drugs as well as the general biochemistry of mental processes. Others follow the tradition of Pavlov and study experimentally induced behavior and laboratory mechanisms for changing it. This led to modern behaviorism, of which B.F. Skinner is the most prominent spokesman. It also laid the ground work for modern experimental psychology. Some have followed Harry Stack Sullivan's lead and study relationships between people. Many have expanded on the explorations of Sigmund Freud who first described the mental mechanisms that linked abnormal behavior to normal behavior.

Students should not worry about which tradition is correct but should appreciate that each of these traditions approach different aspects of mental disorders. A long standing argument which should be dismissed as outdated is the one about whether mental disorders are rooted in psychology or physiology or whether they are due to nature or nurture. Intelligent scientists know that these are not exclusive terms but different aspects of that which is a combination of both. In other words, mental disorders are rooted in both psychology and physiology and are products of both nature and nurture or else they are rooted in neither.

Identifying causes for mental disorders is also complicated by the fact that they are heterogeneous. Investigators over the past one hundred years have expanded what they have been investigating. In the nineteenth century investigators studied disturbed people who clearly were different from normals. They behaved bizarrely; they were paranoid and unmanageable and as it turns out many of them actually were discovered simply to have tertiary syphilis. At that time there were also a group of people who were disturbed who did not have syphilis. Kraeplin identified them as having what later has been called schizophrenia and bipolar illness. Around the same time, Freud described gradations of mental disorders. In other words, people were not simply disturbed or normal, they could also be neurotic or anxious. He also described the little bit of craziness and childishness that "normal" people experience. Today investigators not only study the severe mental disorders, the ones that make people act strangely like schizophrenia or bipolar illness but they also study adjustment disorders, panic attacks, sexual problems, normal mental mechanisms, mild phobias and personality disorders.

Sometimes with all the diagnostic descriptions it is hard for professionals and laymen alike to decide what is normal and what is a disorder. For both investigators and allied health professionals it is important to remember that mental disorders present in specific syndromatic ways; certain diagnostic criteria must be met before a person is diagnosed as having a mental disorder.

## MAJOR TYPES OF MENTAL DISORDERS

There are many types of mental disorders but mental health professionals see only a few major ones in their practices. Without apologizing, I will focus on the mental disorders primarily treated by mental health professionals. This will give you a sense of the kinds of patients that they see in their practices, in psychiatric hospitals, in community mental health clinics and psychiatric units of general hosptials.

### Schizophrenia

Schizophrenia is a major public health problem. Most of the patients in state psychiatric hospitals have schizophrenia, many "bag ladies" and "street people" have schizophrenia, as well as a would-be presidential assassin. It is an important cause of human suffering, loss of productivity and public expense.

In spite of a relatively low number of new cases per year, patients with schizophrenia represent a large number of the total U.S. population, about one percent. The number is so large because the syndrome is essentially a life long condition with an early onset. Rather than multiple sclerosis, schizophrenia is the major crippler of young adults.

Schizophrenia, a term adopted by Bleuler in 1911, means a splitting of the mind. What he wanted to convey with the term is the massive disintegration of emotions, thinking and behavior that occurs during schizophrenic decompensation. Schizophrenics are not persons with split personalities, rather their thinking is poorly integrated with behavior and emotions. Eve in *The Three Faces of Eve* didn't have schizophrenia, she had multiple personalities.

The principle problem with schizophrenics is that their thinking becomes disorganized and illogical when they are troubled or stressed. The illogical and disorganized thought of schizophrenia has certain characteristics. The content and form of the thought is disordered. Thought content refers to what is preoccupying a person. Patients with schizophrenia may become preoccupied with delusions. These are false beliefs on selective and incorrect interpretations of reality. The patient with schizophrenia may have the delusion that others wish to harm him. Magical thinking is also another characteristic disturbance of thought content. For example, schizophrenic patients may believe that they have special powers. They may believe that when they blink people will agree with them or that they control the rising and setting of the sun. The flow of ideas and words or form of the thought may also be disturbed. The thinking may appear choppy, disconnected and loose. Sometimes thinking can be so disconnected that the schizophrenic patient has "word salad." Ideas are tossed out in a seemingly random fashion.

Besides having disordered thought, schizophrenic patients may behave bizarrely and have perceptual disturbances like auditory hallucinations. They may become catatonic, withdrawn, or even violent, but contrary to popular belief, violent behavior occurs in a minority of schizophrenics.

Some investigators refer to the disordered thought, perceptual disturbances and bizarre behaviors as positive symptoms. These are symptoms that were not present before the schizophrenic episode and which often resolve after the flare-up.

Some schizophrenic patients have negative symptoms like indifference, apathy and a lack of emotionality. Patients with these symptoms cannot perform simple tasks; things that most of us take for granted like knowing how to fix a meal or take a bus. These patients are not retarded; they seem to lack volition or will. Many withdrawn, apathetic "street people" or "bag ladies" have these negative symptoms.

There is a tradition of subclassification according to the predominant symptoms. In catatonic schizophrenia, catatonia predominates. In herbephrenic or disorganized schizophrenia, the patient's behavior and thinking is extremely disorganized. Delusions of grandeur or paranoia predominate in paranoid schizophrenia and in undifferentiated schizophrenia the negative symptoms are most noticeable.

Schizophrenic symptoms usually begin in young adults. In some patients the change is dramatic; some patients may have been leaders in school and bright students but when the symptoms begin their thinking and appearance change dramatically. Other schizophrenics, before becoming clearly symptomatic, may have seemed odd or strange to others for many years.

Schizophrenia may follow three courses. The positive symptoms may reoccur sporadically when the patient is troubled; the patients may have a single episode which must last at least six months and then never have another; or the patient may be continuously symptomatic with positive and negative symptoms.

There are some conditions that can mimic schizophrenia. Ingestion of drugs like amphetamine and cocaine can produce a schizophrenic-like picture. Affective or emotional disorders like mania resembles schizophrenia. Toxic of confusional states with combativeness due to hypoxia, uremia, or other metabolic abnormalities may be confused with schizophrenia. In spite of these conditions, experienced clinicians can reliably diagnose schizophrenia by focusing on the course of symptoms, the pattern of symptoms, family history and initial presentation. For the clinician, there are no laboratory tests to confirm the diagnosis although radiological techniques and certain biochemical markers are promising. Presently, the diagnosis of schizophrenia is exclusively a clinical one.

Treatment of these patients has changed dramatically over the past 25 years largely due to deinstitutionalization, a social policy aimed at lowering the census of state mental hospitals. In the past, patients with schizophrenia remained in psychiatric hospitals most of their lives. Now, for a variety of reasons, schizophrenics are treated primarily as outpatients with periodic hospitalization. Comprehensive outpatient programs attempt to alleviate both positive and negative symptoms. Medication controls the positive symptoms of schizophrenia and a variety of treatment approaches such as vocational and social skills training, and partial hospitalization help to overcome the negative symtoms. In spite of these programs, recurrence rates are high. Patients usually are hospitalized when agitation, auditory hallucinations and bizarre behavior cause them to endanger themselves or others. Treatment will improve as health care professionals develop comprehensive, consistent treatment for these patients (3).


## Affective Disorders

Affective disorders are a group of psychiatric conditions in which a disturbance of mood rather than thought predominate. Affect, as in the term affective, refers to how patients display their mood. If a patient is depressed and his affect fits his mood, he will frown, sigh, cry, slump in his chair, appear unkept and sad. If he has all of these features then he is considered to have a depressed affect.

The diagnosis, major depression, depends upon the presence of a constellation of signs and symptoms predominated by depressed affect and by feelings of sadness and despondency. There are also associated symptoms which can cause significant occupational and social disability. Patients may become agitated and irritable or they may conversely become withdrawn and solemn. They may neglect hygiene, stop eating properly and become preoccupied with somatic complaints, visiting doctor after doctor. In severe cases, auditory hallucinations and somatic delusions may occur; often but not inevitably both hallucinations and delusions will fit the mood. Severely depressed patients may have hallucinations that are self-deprecatory, voices telling them that they are worthless and they may also have the delusions that their bodies are rotting and wasting away. Patients with these symptoms resemble schizophrenics, especially if they are agitated. Others, especially elder patients, may seem senile and absent-minded.

A large number of people have chronic life-long intermittent depressions. The associated symptoms in these patients, if they occur at all, are not as severe as in major depression. Just about everyone after significant losses feels depressed; this is usually short-lived and clearly related to the loss. Moderate to severe depression of mood which is persistent and inappropriate to the occasion should be considered pathological.

Patients with both major depression and manic episodes have bipolar illness. These patients vacillate between the two poles of euphoria and despondency; depression and mania. When manic, they seem full of energy, but they often have associated symptoms which cause them trouble. The euphoria may change to restlessness, irritability and distractability. Their elation may lead to grandiosity and then to frank delusions of grandiosity. They may get involved in activities that have a high potential for painful consequences, such as investing in unwise business ventures or being sexually indiscreet.

As with schizophrenia, diagnosing affective disorders depends upon the clinical exam. There are no lab or radiological tests which can confirm the diagnosis. Clinicians must anticipate that drugs, endocrine disorders and metabolic disturbances may cause depressive or manic symptoms. Often persons with medical illnesses such as diabetes and heart failure will have pervasive and persistent depression because they are sick and debilitated.

The treatment of affective disorders has improved over the last 30 years. Psychotherapeutic approaches of the 1930s and 1940s have been enhanced and suppressed by chemotherapy. Psychological treatments provide support and help patients to improve coping skills. Psychotherapy is the main intervention for mild to moderate chronic depressions, but when patients are severely depressed or manic, psychotherapy has been less than satisfactory. Drugs such as lithium carbonate for bipolar illness and anti-depressants for major depressions have effectively reduced the acute symptoms of these disorders. Improvement usually occurs within several weeks while maintenance treatment helps to prevent recurrence of symptoms. Electroconvulsive treatment, in spite of its bad reputation, is an extremely effective treatment for individuals who cannot tolerate medications or who have not responded to them (4).

## Anxiety Disorders

Anxiety is an unpleasant feeling similar to fear. Anxiety, like fear, causes muscular tension, restlessness, tremor, excessive perspiration, rapid pulse and hyperventilation. Chronic anxiety may cause fatigue, insomnia, irritability, poor concentration and dysphoria. Anxiety may also occur episodically. When anxiety occurs in the presence of specific objects like dogs or in places like elevators or high places, this is called a phobia. Panic attacks are another form of anxiety. Patients with these attacks have air hunger, palpitations and hyperventilation.

Psychotherapy is the treatment of choice for chronic anxiety, while behavioral therapy, anxiolytics, and antidepressants are best for panic attacks and some phobias. The anxiolytics, drugs that are specifically able to reduce anxiety, have only become available in the last thirty years (5).

## Drug Abuse

A number of substances and drugs with powerful psychological effects have come into use during the past 15 years. Heroin use has increased steadily and current estimates of daily heroin users range from 200,000 to 800,000. Stimulants and sedatives are even more widely used.

The major drugs of misuse that bring patients to mental health professionals are the opiates, the sedative/hypnotics and the stimulants. Problems related to the use of hallucinogens and inhalants are less common today but still occur and can be dangerous.

The direct toxic effects of the drug and withdrawal syndromes bring patients to the clinician's attention. The toxic effects are due to the physiological and psychological properties of the drug especially when too much is taken. Panic attacks, irritability, and impaired judgments are common toxic effects. Severe toxic effects due to drug overdosage include apnea, hypotension, cardiac arrest and other complications. Sedative/hypnotic overdosage followed by heroin overdosage are leading causes of death in young adults between 19 and 25. Chronic stimulant abuse as well as overdosage causes symptoms similar to schizophrenia.

Withdrawal syndromes also bring patients to clinicians. The affects of abrupt cessation of stimulants like amphetamines and cocaine may cause profound depression and lassitude. Abrupt opiate withdrawal may cause discomfort similar to a severe case of the flu, but not life threatening. The withdrawal syndrome from sedative drugs is very dangerous causing seizures, tremulousness, confusion and death.

PCP or phencyclidine is another drug of concern to clinicians. It was introduced in the late 50s as a potential intravenous anesthetic but the side effects led to a cessation of usage in humans. The drug when taken produces both central nervous system stimulation and depression. These effects are related to dosage. Toxic drug effects consist of severe agitation, excitement, and even schizophrenic–like sypmtoms. In extremely high dosages coma and seizures may occur.

A variety of hallucinogens, such as LSD, DMT, and mescaline, can produce confusion, hallucinations, and panic reactions or "bad trips." Marijuana continues to be the most widely used drug in our society other than tobacco, alcohol, and caffeine. Although there are no abstinence syndromes or toxic reactions with marijuana per se, there are troublesome side affects. Panic reactions, paranoia and delusions can occur. Most troubling of all, apathy, indifference, and lack of motivation may occur when the drug is used chronically.

Drug abuse like most mental disorders is chronic, recurrent and persistent. It requires consistent, comprehensive treatment because there are no quick fixes. Short–term, intensive programs seldom work over the long haul. Usually treatment involves three phases. First, the drug abuser must be detoxified. This involves giving patients equivalent dosages of a similar drug and then gradually tapering it. The second phase involves treatment of coping difficulties which finally merges into the third phase of rehabilitation in which the person works in a structured program free of drugs (6).

## Alcohol Abuse

Alcoholism occurs when drinking of alcoholic beverages adversely effects a person's general health, vocational or social adjustment. Alcoholics may drink either episodically or habitually. Symptoms of alcoholism vary from patient to patient, but generally the condition proceeds in stages. During the prodromal stage, "social" drinking is maintained, but tolerance to alcohol increases. Larger amounts of alcohol are required to produce intoxication and irritation to the gastrointestinal track. Occasional drunkeness may occur in settings where it is tolerated. During the early symptomatic phase, there is definite dependence and increased drinking. Drinking occurs daily and if alcohol is omitted there is likely to be irritability. The drinker may avoid situations where alcohol is not served or may drink directly before or after these occasions. Family and social life begins to suffer because of increased absenteeism and irritability. During the advanced symptomatic phase, dependence on alcohol increases while tolerance decreases. The drinker is often intoxicated and may experience "blackouts" or periods of amnesia. Arrests for drunken driving and public intoxication occur during this phase. Jobs are lost and family life also deteriorates. In the terminal phase, the physiological consequences of chronic consumption predominates.

The liver is the organ most significantly damaged by chronic alcohol ingestion. Alcohol abuse also interferes with metabolism and contributes to deficiency of vitamins. It alters numerous functions of the endocrine system and has been implicated in impotency and in early onset of menopause and amenorrhea. Chronic abuse affects the cardiovascular system including a specific cardiomyopathy and mild to moderate hypertension. Brain dysfunction has been esetimated in 50 to 70 percent of detoxified alcoholics while the risk of cancer of the tongue, mouth, and throat as well as the esophagus, larynx and liver is increased in alcoholics. It has been associated with birth defects especially the fetal alcohol syndrome which is characterized by a specific cluster of facial abnormalities and defective growth rates.

Diagnosis of alcoholism is based on history and physical exam. An accurate history is difficult to obtain because many alcoholics in the advanced stages disavow or minimize their habit. Besides interviewing the patient the clinician should also speak to family members. Important questions to ask are — How do you use alcohol? Has it gotten you into trouble before? The interviewer must pay careful attention to how the patient responds. Is the patient evasive? Does he or she protest too much? Several lab tests may increase your level of suspicion. For example, elevated alcohol level in the serum without obvious signs of intoxication is a diagnostic finding. Certain batteries of metabolic tests, liver function tests, and red blood cells indices may assist but cannot confirm the diagnosis.

Treatment begins with recognition of this disorder. Often the patient is not told of the diagnosis or clinical suspicion until the condition is far advanced. The diagnosis and treatment recommendation should not be kept from the patient because of clinicians' fears of offending or frightening him. Most patients in the advanced stages require hospitalization for detoxification and treatment of associated problems. In the early stages, alcoholics may be treated as outpatients with psychotherapy. Referral to Alcoholics Anonymous may meet the needs of some patients as well as treatment with the medication, antibuse.

There are about 10 million problem drinkers, including men and women, suffering from alcoholism in the United States. In addition, there are about 3 million problem drinkers among youth. Other surveys indicate that 7 percent of adults and 19 percent of youths experience problems with alcohol. Alcohol abuse and alcoholism cost the United States billions of dollars per year. It is commonly implicated in injuries and deaths which occur in home, industrial, recreational and motor vehicle accidents. It has been implicated in many crimes and has been related to the formation of criminal behavior because of the disinhibition and excessive violence that it may cause (7).

## Mental Retardation

Although I.Q. numbers are used to differentiate severity, mental retardation is not simply a deficit in intellectual functioning. Definitions of mental retardation emphasize more than mental subnormality; for a person to be considered mentally retarded he must also be socially handicapped and developmentally impaired. The symptoms must persist into adulthood and are largely incurable. This definition is especially applicable to severe mental retardation. Persons with mjld retardation may meet the criteria at one time and not at another. In some situations, they may perform adequately while in others they may fail. This is especially true of persons with mild intellectual deficits who are in school.

Specific causes for mild retardation such as damage to the central nervous system are seldom identified. Most of the cases of mild retardation are thought to be due to "environmental deprivation." Severe cases usually have identifiable causes such as chromosal abnormalities, and central nervous system trauma or anoxia at birth (1).

## Mental Disorders in Children

Delays in normal development, emotional disorders and conduct disorders account for most of the mental health problems in children. About 5 to 15 percent of children between 3 and 15 have problems such as these. Emotional disorders consist of anxiety, depression and pre–occupation with somatic complaints. Conduct disorders include poor peer relations, running away, theft and aggressiveness. Abnormalities in development may occur in speech, social, psychosexual, motor, sensory and emotional areas.

Certain syndromes arise only in childhood. Infantile autism is a rare condition in which there is a pervasive impairment in the child's ability to interact with persons. Stereotyped behaviors and mental retardation may occur with this syndrome. Another group of childhood syndromes are the attention deficit disorders. These disorders may occur with or without hyperactivity and consist of poor control of behavior, short attention span, extreme excitability and impairment in relationships with others. Another group of disorders are the learning disabilities. A child may be unable to learn in the classroom because of difficulties perceiving, integrating, retaining or transmitting words. Conditions such as schizophrenia and the affective disorders also occur in children.

Emotional disorders in children may result from physical abnormalities, inadequate parenting or traumatic events that interfere with the development. Often, the emotional disorders are forerunners of difficulty in adult life. For example, chidlren with the attention deficit disorders have increased rates of delinquency and sociopathy when they become adults. Conduct disorders often are chronic and eventually evolve into personaltiy disorders (1).

## Mental Disorders of the Elderly

Today, over 10 percent of the population are over 65 and by the year 2000 it is projected that nearly 15 percent of the population will be over this age. Today, most of the elderly are taking care of themselves in their own homes. Individuals residing in nursing homes tend to be 80 years or over and represent a minority of the total elderly.

The major mental disorder of old age is senile dementia, a syndrome characterized by a severe loss of social and intellectual functioning including memory and the ability to abstract. This is a condition of the brain tissue and is not simply "hardening of the arteries." In hospitalized geriatric patients it is a common condition, while in the community it is uncommon. The elderly are also susceptible to confusional states or delirium. The disorientation and agitation of delirium can be caused by many factors including fever, electrolyte abnormalities and most commonly drug misuse. Many physicians are not sensitized to this population's decreased tolerance to drugs and often elderly patients see many physicians who may prescribe different drugs.

The mental disorders of childhood and young adulthood often persist into old age. The proportion of aged persons with schizophrenia and affective disorders has been rising. Major depression is an important problem for the elderly especially among those isolated in the community and institutions. Depression may sometimes mimic senile dementia and in fact the term pseudo-dementia is given to patients who have this syndrome (1).

## CONCLUSIONS

Patients with mental disorders share several characteristics. They have symptoms which cause them distress and disability. These symptoms occur in specific patterns and follow a course over time. Patients with mental disorders are often stigmatized and found blameworthy. These patients tend to suffer from their symptoms for a long time because most mental disorders are chronic or subacute with a high rate of recurrence. Ultimate causes for mental disorders have not been identified because most are multidetermined. Finally, most patients with mental disorders get better with treatment and therapy but seldom quickly and dramatically.

## REFERENCES

1. Report to the President: President's Commission on Mental Health, Vol. 1. Washington, DC: Superintendent of Documents, 1978.

2. American Psychiatric Association: Diagnostic and Statistical Manual of Mental Disorders (Third Edition). Washington, DC: American Psychiatric Association, 1980.

3.Carpenter WT, Strauss JS: Schizophrenia. New York: Plenum Medical Book Co., 1981.

4. Val R, Gaviria M, Flaherty JA: Affective Disorders: Psychopathology and Treatment. Chicago: Year Book Medical, 1982.

5. Rosenbaum JF: Current concepts in psychiatry: The drug treatment of anxiety. New Eng J Med, 306:401-404, 1982.

6. Khantzian EJ, McKenna GJ: Acute toxic and withdrawal reactions associated with drug use and abuse. Ann Int Med, 90:361-372, 1979.

7. Eckardtmu, Harford TC, Kaelber CT, *et al.*: Health hazards associated with alcohol consumption. JAMA, 246:648-667, 1981.

# Chapter 2

<br>

INTERVIEWING TECHNIQUES:
MENTAL HEALTH PROBLEMS CAN PRESENT ANYWHERE

DARYL K. KNOX, M.D.
GEORGE L. ADAMS, M.D.

Health care providers are constantly told throughout their training, that understanding their patients as whole human beings rather than thinking of them as "diseases" is of utmost importance. However, until very recently, little attention has been focused on how to acquire this understanding in the training of health professionals. Training curricula usually devote inadequate instruction on dealing with a patient's emotions. This situation is truly unfortunate as health care providers will often have interactions with patients where feelings and emotions are expressed. It is not surprising that being ill, or hospitalized, is fertile ground from which emotional problems come to the surface. The skills necessary for health care providers to be of benefit to patients when feelings and emotions arise can indeed be learned. One way to obtain these skills is through mastering good interviewing techniques. Although many encounters with patients will take place outside of a formal interview setting, the skills essential to good interviewing should still be applied in day-to-day patient caregiver interactions. These interactions can occur in the clinic, in the laboratory, in the x-ray department, or in any part of the hospital where patients have contact with health care providers. To this end, the skills taught in basic diagnostic interviewing allow one to focus on how to establish a more positive interaction with patients. This chapter will examine some of these important skills.

## THE INTERVIEW

It is fundamental for health care providers to acquire good interviewing skills. Interviewing is an important method by which information that is vital to the care of the patient is gathered.

Often, an accurate diagnosis and effective treatment plan depends on the information one has obtained from interviewing the patient. However, interviewing involves more than just information gathering. It is an interaction between individuals. This interaction not only yields significant data, but also alleviates anxiety, and at times influences or alters behavior (1). Sometimes the interaction between the patient and the health care provider contributes as much to the patient's recovery as the provision of the correct treatment plan. Therefore, learning appropriate interviewing techniques is helpful in developing a positive as well as therapeutic interaction between the health care provider and the patient. For the allied health and nursing professional who is not involved in mental health care provision, the most important interviewing skills to master are obtaining an accurate medical history, observing behavioral and emotional clues that may suggest that the patient is anxious, and learning interventions that help to alleviate anxiety or emotional distress. Within the mental health field, the interview assumes even more of a central role. In many instances it can serve as a treatment modality (such as, the beginning of psychotherapy) in addition to being a diagnostic tool.

Indeed, mental health problems can present anywhere within the health care continuum. Entry into the health care system places most persons under tremendous stress. The fear of illness and pain contribute greatly to the patients' anxiety. This anxiety can be exhibited in a number of ways, from the patient being withdrawn, quiet, and overly compliant, all the way to his being demanding, rude, and uncooperative. At times, no matter what the care providers' role is in the treatment of the patient, an intervention may be necessary or appropriate in order to facilitate the patient's eventual recovery.

Bernstein and Dana (2) emphasize the importance of the words and gestures used by health care providers in determining the success or failure of treatment. They also stress the importance of emotional factors upon physical illness (1). The authors will focus on the skills necessary to make the appropriate interventions to deal with the patients' feelings when mental health issues arise.

## INTERVIEWING SKILLS

The process of interviewing and interacting with patients on an interpersonal level leaves many health care providers feeling anxious and uncertain of just how this level of understanding and enhanced communication is attained. Thus, the attitudes towards interviewing skills range from seeing it as a natural gift that few people possess, to the other extreme of seeing it as nothing more than interacting as one would in a social setting (1). Neither of these viewpoints is appropriate.

Perhaps the most important ingredients necessary for good interviewing are the ability to communicate clearly, to listen well, to observe accurately, and to be empathic (2, 3). Having these skills enable the health professional to build the patients confidence by conveying an attitude of competence and of genuine interest in the patient and his or her concerns. Each of these skills will be examined in greater detail.

### Communicating Clearly

One of the more basic and essential skills for fostering the relationship and interaction between a patient and health care provider is the ability to communicate in a clear, unambiguous manner. The patient must be able to understand what is being said. So often, health professionals forget that the terms they use daily are often highly technical and have no meaning to the majority of people outside the health field. The use of "medical jargon" can further increase the patient's anxiety. It could lead to misunderstanding, to unwarranted fear and to feelings of inadequacy on the part of the patient. In many cases, patients may not understand what is being said and are too embarrassed to ask for clarification. They often feel they are expected to be knowledgeable and will be perceived as ignorant if they asked questions. This feeling on the part of the patient could prevent him from getting the necessary clarification that could alleviate any fear or anxiety. Thus, it becomes imperative for the health care provider not to impede a therapeutic interaction and rapport by using highly technical language.

The following example, although somewhat exaggerated, illustrates the problems that can ensue from not communicating clearly.

> Mr. Johnson is a 67-year-old retired janitor who was admitted to the hospital to help find the cause of his fainting spells and headaches. His last hospitalization occurred 40 years ago when he had his appendix removed. The following encounter was with a CAT scan technician who had just recently finished training.
>
> *Health Professional:* Mr. Johnson, I see you're here for your CAT Scan.
>
> *Mr. Johnson:* CAT Scan? They told me I was coming to get an x-ray of my head.
>
> *Health Professional:* Well, this is more than just an x-ray machine. it takes tomograms of your brain.
>
> *Mr. Johnson:* To-to-tomograms of the head! They think I have tumors in my head?
>
> *Health Professional:* No, no Mr. Johnson. This is Computerized Axial Tomography. It takes fractions of a millimeter cross-sectional slices of your head. The image is enhanced by the computer, using the difference in the densities of the structures in your cranium.
>
> *Mr. Johnson:* (Looking bewildered, confused, and more depressed) Oh — I see.

It is highly unlikely that Mr. Johnson understood any of the above information. The health profesional failed to take into account the fact that Mr. Johnson probably knew nothing about CAT scans which is a relatively recent x-ray device. One can also assume that Mr. Johnson was concerned about his condition and perhaps fearful of this new procedure. "Is it going to be painful?" "Is there risk involved?" "Will they find something wrong?" These are, perhaps, a few of the questions running through Mr. Johnson's mind. Even though the physician or nurse may have explained the procedure to him earlier, it is not unusual for patients to forget what they have been told when they are ill or under the stress of hospitalization.

Health caregivers should expect to have to repeat instructions or information to their patients. In the above example, the haughty air of the health professional's explanation left Mr. Johnson feeling put-down and inadequate. It closed the door to his asking more questions or getting better clarification of the procedure.

The results are that Mr. Johnson feels more depressed, anxious, fearful and further alienated from his health care providers. A more appropriate interaction would be as follows:

> *Health Professional:* Good morning, Mr. Johnson. I'll be taking your CAT scan.
>
> *Mr. Johnson:* CAT Scan, I thought I was getting an x-ray of my head.
>
> *Health Professional:* That's correct, it is an x-ray of the head. But this machine, using a computer, is able to take more pictures and better pictures so that your doctor can determine with better accuracy what the problems are, if any.
>
> *Mr. Johnson:* The machine looks so big and it sounds like I'll be getting a lot of x-rays.
>
> *Health Professional:* It is a big machine — but surprisingly the amount of radiation used is about the same amount used for a regular x-ray. I've had a lot of people express the same concern.
>
> *Mr. Johnson:* Well, is there any pain involved? I've gone through so many tests in the last 2 days.
>
> *Health Professional:* I can understand your concern, no one likes painful tests. I'm glad to tell you this test involves no pain whatsoever and takes about 30 minutes to finish.
>
> *Mr. Johnson:* That certainly is a relief.

In the above example the health professional explained the procedure in non-technical terms, he acknowledged the appropriateness of Mr. Johnson's questions and feelings, in a way that did not make him feel put-down. The ability to clearly communicate information enhances the interaction and can help decrease a patient's anxiety.


## Listening Effectively

Listening is a very important interview technique and skill, that is often taken for granted. Although the idea of listening sounds easy, it is a difficult skill that requires practice and patience. It is so easy to become preoccupied with one's own thoughts or duties, that a lot of what others are saying is missed. Inability to listen can lead one to assume they know what the patient is saying before he finishes speaking. Stereotypic answers and premature advice are often given. At times there is a tendency to talk too much, which prevents the patient from effectively voicing his concern or feelings.

A tremendous amount of information can be learned from just listening to the patient. Allowing the patient to state his perception of the problem is important. It gives health care providers some understanding of the patient's expectations, worries, or concerns. The expectations may or may not be realistic, but they could be a lot different than one assumes. These differences in expectation if not discussed can lead to mutual misunderstanding. Also worries and concerns are not always directly expressed, therefore one must learn to listen "between the lines," that is, to what is not being said, or what in addition may be implied by the words.

An attentive attitude is also very important. The patient should feel that he is important and has the full attention of the health care provider for all interactions. An atmosphere of being unhurried, and of having as few interruptions as possible should be maintained.

Good listening skills impart to the patient a feeling of importance, and that his concerns are worth considering, and most importantly that someone understands. Gerrard, *et al.* (3) discuss four essential skills of listening. They include: *Passive Listening*, which is remaining silent while patient is talking — allowing him to describe his feelings and concern without interruption. *Acknowledgment Responses*, that is using vocal responses like "uh-huh," and head nods that impart to the patient that you are interested and are listening to what he says. *Encouragers*, this involves using words or phrases like "Please continue," "Tell me more," or "What happened then?" *Active Listening*, or the process of communicating back to the patient in your own words what you think he is saying or feeling. Of the four skills listed, this one is the most important for establishing rapport with the patient. The following clinical example will highlight these suggestions.

A patient has just been informed by her doctor that she has a kidney infection and must be put on IV antibiotics. The nurse comes in shortly therafter to start the intravenous line.

*Patient:* (Smiling nervously) Boy, that needle certainly looks long. I never have liked getting stuck.

*Nurse:* Just hold your arm out, this won't take long. (Ignoring, not acknowledging the patient's fears.)

*Patient:* The thought of having this needle in my arm for such a long time bothers me. My aunt had such a problem with hers, it kept coming out.

> *Nurse:* Well, she was probably moving her arm about carelessly and pulled it out. Please keep still while I try to find a vein.
> *Patient:* She finally ended up getting a real bad infection in her arm probably because the IV was in her arm so long. Ouch!
> *Nurse:* There, I told you it wouldn't take long.

In this situation, the nurse demonstrated poor listening skills and appeared to be disinterested in understanding the patient. He was more preoccupied with starting the IV. During this interaction the patient was interrupted, ignored, and her concerns and fears were not acknowledged. The nurse also failed to actively listen and reflect to the patient his understanding of her concerns. The impact of this encounter upon the patient could result in her feeling more concerned or anxious about having an IV in her arm. She may even become angry and refuse to have this necessary treatment. If handled more appropriately by the nurse, the interaction and rapport with the patient could be more positive. Let's look at how it might have occurred differently.

> *Patient:* Boy, that needle certainly looks long. I never liked getting stuck!
> *Nurse:* You're worried that it might be painful.
> *Patient:* That's right. Plus the fact that it stays in your arm so long. My aunt had such problems with hers, it kept coming out and she ended up getting an infection in her arm.
> *Nurse:* I can certainly understand your concern. You're probably frightened that you might have some complications from this IV.
> *Patient:* Well. I am a little nervous about it. My aunt still has a scar on her arm from it.
> *Nurse:* It sounds like she had a pretty rough time. I'm glad you told me about that, because having experienced that with your aunt, most people would be nervous. I'll be glad to answer any questions you have about your IV and you can be assured that we are taking every precaution to try to prevent complications.
> *Patient:* Thank you, that really makes me feel better.

## Observing Accurately

Good observation skills enable health care providers to add a lot more information, beyond what the patient tells them. What patients do not say is often just as important a clue to underlying feelings as what they say. By observing facial expression, mannerisms and behaviors along with the verbal content, valuable insight into the patients feelings and emotional state can be obtained, especially if there is an inconsistency between behavior and verbal content.

There is often a tendency on the part of patients to deny or minimize their worries or concerns. However, their behavior in the form of nervous twitching, a sad expression, or a tremulous voice often belie their verbal response of "everything is fine." This situation can provide an excellent opportunity for the health care provider to intervene and lessen the anxiety with such patients. A patient's facial expression or affect is particularly important to note for it gives valuable clues to what is going on. Benjamin Pope (4) states that "as an instrument of communication, the major function of the face is the expression of emotion." He goes on to cite another current author who presents evidence that supports Charles Darwin's beliefs that human facial expression is a biologically derived process through evolution. This is to say that there are certain facial expressions such as anger, fear, sadness or joy that are universal and usually recognizable even across cultural lines (4).

The above could prove helpful when one encounters a patient who tightly grips the arms of his stretcher or wheelchair and has a frightened look on his face prior to a procedure. Rather than ignoring these emotional cues and going ahead with the procedure, acknowledgment of the patient's distress and inquiry into his concerns would be in order. The following case example illustrates how this might happen.

> *Physician's Assistant:* Hello, Mr. Nelson, my name is Gloria, I'll be assisting Dr. Rodriquez with your protoscope exams.
>
> *Patient:* (Clutching arm of wheelchair tighter, and looking tense) Hi.
>
> *Physician's Assistant:* Have you ever had a protoscope exam before?
>
> *Patient:* No, I haven't, but Dr. Rodriguez told me a little bit about it.
>
> *Physician's Assistant:* I'll be happy to answer any further questions you might have.
>
> *Patient:* (Shakes head and mumbles softly) No, I have no questions.

> *Physician's Assistant:* It's not unusual for people to feel nervous before this procedure. I wonder if you might have some concerns that I could help you with.
>
> *Patient:* (Looking somewhat relieved) Well, maybe I am a little nervous. I've heard so much about these exams from friends who have had one. . . about them being so painful. My roommate told me its the worst experience he has ever had.
>
> *Physician's Assistant:* Well, I can certainly understand your concern. Most of the people who come through here have voiced similar concerns. While I can't guarantee you that you won't feel any discomfort — I can tell you a little more about what to expect and how we try to minimize the discomfort.

In this example, the physician's assistant took into account the patient's concern over the upcoming procedure by observing his behavior. In a non–judgmental and supportive manner, she was able to get the patient to talk about his concerns. Without discounting the fact that the procedure can be uncomfortable, she was willing to give the patient an opportunity to voice his concerns. At the same time, the physician's assistant was able to inform the patient about what he could expect during the procedure and to reassure him that they were willing to do all that was possible to minimize the discomfort. As a result, Mr. Nelson was a lot less tense and apprehensive. As he became more relaxed, he was more cooperative and made the procedure a lot easier to perform.

## Being Empathic

Empathy is the ability to understand a patient's feelings or perceptions. To be able to see and experience an emotion or an issue from the other's point of view is fundamentally important for building trust and rapport between the patient and health care provider. The ability to put oneself into the patient's shoes does not necessarily mean you have to agree or go along with whatever the patient tells you. Sometimes a patient's feelings or perceptions may be based on erroneous information or faulty reasoning. Being empathic implies that one is able to impart to the other person, that one truly understands his or her concern, and does not judge their feelings as being either inappropriate or wrong.

Everyone at some point in their life has experienced emotions of being sad, angry, anxious, or frightened. It is partly from our own experiences with these feelings and emotions that we acquire the ability to be empathic. Often, these strong emotions and feelings are not easy to handle and cause discomfort. Due to the nature of their work, health care providers frequently encounter these feelings in their patients. The usual tendency is to minimize, ignore, or deny the patient the reality of his perceptions. Sometimes this happens because the patient's emotions trigger some memory in the health care provider of his own discomfort in handling that type of feeling.

As stated earlier, patients in a medical setting are usually under stress by virtue of the fact that they are ill. This being the case, it is inappropriate to cover up these feelings or emotions when they arise. The responses that health care providers give when patients express these emotions or concerns must be carefully considered. Bernstein and Bernstein (5) categorize the verbal responses in health care provider and patient interventions into five basic types: evaluative, hostile, reassuring, probing, and understanding.

The evaluative response is highly judgmental and has the effect of invalidating the patient's feelings and implies what he should or ought to feel. A hostile response not only diminishes the validity of a patient's feeling but also puts the patient down by implying some negative characteristic such as immaturity or ignorance. For instance, if a patient says "I really don't like needles stuck in my arm, they really hurt," a hostile reply would be, "Nonsense! It's just a little prick, you shouldn't be such a big baby." The reassuring response is also inappropriate because it denies the patient the right to feel the way he does, "Now, now I can understand that you're upset but don't worry, everything will be alright soon." With the probing response, by asking rapid fire questions, the health provider leaves the impression that if the patient will only give more information some solution will eventually be found to solve his problems. The understanding response is a much more empathic response; it communicates to the patient that his point of view is understood. This response conveys that his feelings and emotions can be discussed in a non-judgmental manner.

Empathy is one of the most important skills or techniques health care providers can possess for establishing positive and therapeutic interactions with their patients. The ability to be empathic draws upon one's personal experiences and background. Being empathic also utilizes skills that can be learned. It requires all the aforementioned skills of communicating clearly, attentive listening, observing and being understanding in one's responses. It also requires looking for the hidden meanings, and not just the verbal content of what that patient is saying. It is often these hidden meanings that address the patient's feelings and concern.

The following exchange occurs between a patient, who has just recently been told he has diabetes, and the hospital nutritionist. During the course of discussing his new dietary regimine the patient angrily remarks: "My doctor tells me, all of a sudden, I have diabetes and then all of these specialists appear. Everyone is telling me how I should now do this and change the way I do that! Now here you are telling me what I *can* and *cannot* eat. I hate all of these new rules and regulations." In this interaction, rather than becoming defensive or angry, an empathic and understanding response by the nutritionist could have been: "Naturally you are concerned about having diabetes and it is upsetting and worrisome to you not knowing what impact it might have on your lifestyle."

With this response, the patient is made to feel that he is understood. Also he knows that the nutritionist is concerned, and also willing and comfortable with exploring his feelings.

## DIFFICULT PATIENTS

It has already been stated that the ill, hospitalized patient is under stress. This stress can be due to the fears that accompany illness, "What is wrong with me? Will I need surgery? Will I be all right? Am I going to die?" The fear of pain and death are common concerns of hospitalized patients. Anxiety can also stem from being in the strange environment of a hospital with all the different health care personnel, unfamiliar equipment and the hurried, hectic pace. The patient usually becomes subject to new rules and regulations, lack of privacy, and "assaults" upon their bodies. These normal hospital routines and regulations can leave patients feeling helpless, totally dependent, frustrated, scared or angry. Since everyone handles stress in their  own special way, some patients handle stress in more socially adaptable ways than do others. There are some patients who have very limited abilities to deal with stress, and tend to respond in a very predictable, stereotypic manner when any stress is encountered. This latter type of patient is unlikely to change a lifetime of behavior in one hospitalization no matter how empathically their health care providers respond. The angry–hostile patient, the paranoid–suspicious patient, and the depressed patient can be particularly challenging to health care providers. Utilizing the intervention skills mentioned earlier, we will now focus on strategies that may be helpful in establishing rapport with these more difficult patients.

## The Angry Patient

At some point in their career, every health professional will encounter the angry or hostile patient. These patients can be quite provocative, and can cause one to respond in a likewise angry fashion. However, when the health professional responds with anger, the situation usually is made worse. The most important thing is to maintain one's composure. Allow the patient to ventilate their anger and find out specifically the patient's concerns. It is important to understand the nature of the problem from the patient's perspective. One should try to explore the feelings that may be underlying the patient's anger. It is "only by becoming more aware and developing more understanding of a patient's feelings can the doctor react more therapeutically to patients" (5). Furthermore, in order to be helpful to the angry patient, the health care professional must be aware of his own angry feelings and impulses.

In the following example the above points are illustrated.

> *Patient:* (On a stretcher in x-ray waiting room) — (angrily) "What the hell is going on here? I've been waiting here 2 hours. Can't you people work any faster? You probably just don't give a damn about other folks' time."
>
> *Health Professional:* I'm sorry you've had to wait sir, two hours is a long time to wait.
>
> *Patient:* You're damn right, it is a long time.
>
> *Health Professional:* (Feeling defensive) We are short staffed and trying to work as fast as we can. Please try to be more considerate and . . .
>
> *Patient:* (Interrupting and becoming louder) Well the amount I'm gonna get billed for all these so-called "tests" I would expect

you all would work a little faster. Anyway, I don't like your attitude — Who is your supervisor?

By allowing himself to become angry and defensive, the health professional in this example only added fuel to the fire. Perhaps if he had been more aware of his own anger toward this patient he may have been better able to allow the patient to ventilate his concerns. There are certainly many reasons for a patient to be legitimately angry. Things can go wrong in a hospital such as delays in getting lab and diagnostic work done, menu foul-ups or even inappropriate or insensitive remarks by the staff. Sometimes the anger is not expressed directly, where it should be. It is displayed on to someone who is more accessible, less threatening, or who just happens to be in the right place at the wrong time. Often, this anger is a defense against some underlying fear or anxiety. It can be the patient's attempt to fight back and gain some control over an environment or illness that has left him feeling helpless.

When the patient becomes angry, it is important to remain calm. If the patient's history is known, it may shed some light on why the patient may react that way. Do not become defensive or apologetic, but let the patient ventilate his feelings. Attempt to clarify and then to understand the patient's feelings. Also realize that not all situations can be satisfactorily resolved. Some patients will become obnoxious, insulting, and even more hostile despite any reasonable attempts to address their concerns. Satisfaction should be obtained in the feeling that one has tried to be helpful. Unnecessary abuse, however, should not be tolerated. One may need to convey to the patient that he will not be allowed to publicly humiliate or embarrass you for no apparent reason. Even in this situation, it is important to maintain a tactful and professional composure.

## The Suspicious Patient

When one encounters the overly suspicious or paranoid patient, it must be kept in mind that the underlying dynamic of these patients is usually feelings of inadequacy or unworthiness (7). They harbor feelings that the world is against them and everyone wants to do them harm. Avoidance and resistance of any intrusion upon their inner feelings is their primary goal. Thus, in a hospital setting where lack of privacy, personal questions and intimate contact with the body are the norm, anxiety and paranoid defenses are at their peak in patients with paranoid personality traits.

With the paranoid or suspicious patient, it is important to respect their desire to remain emotionally distant. Intrusive questions or attempts to establish rapport too quickly must be avoided, or the patient is likely to misjudge your intentions. It is important to be honest and sincere in all encounters. Explain thoroughly each procedure to the patient beforehand. Paranoid patients are particularly keen at sensing anxiety, anger or other emotions of those around them. It is important to acknowledge one's own feelings if the patient senses them and to correct any misunderstanding the patient may have about your motives. For example, if a patient should comment that you appear tired or angry and that assessment is accurate, acknowledge the patient's perspectiveness and if appropriate give an explanation. Otherwise the patient may wrongly assume the feelings are directed towards him. Also, arguing with the suspicious patient is to be avoided as it may agitate him unnecessarily (8).

## The Depressed Patient

Depression is common enough that undoubtedly every allied health professional will at some time in their career experience a patient who is depressed. Usually it is a natural occurrence with anyone experiencing a significant medical illness or hospitalization. Patients who are severely depressed and/or suicidal should be hospitalized and treated on a psychiatric unit. In other settings, depressed patients may present in a variety of ways. They may appear sad with an expressionless face, be uncommunicative, withdrawn, irritable or extremely helpless and dependent. The most important thing is to maintain a positive, supportive stance. Commenting on the patients' sad expression may sometimes open the door to the patients' verbalizing and sharing their feelings. Listen empathically, avoid giving advice or false reassurance. Sometimes depressed patients have a tendency to catastrophize or make things sound much worse than they appear. Circular, negative thinking is also quite common. It is important to emphasize the positive and gently challenge the patients' negative observation if you know they are not accurate. For example, if a patient responds to "How are you feeling today?" with "I feel lousy, I don't think I'm ever going to be better." It may be helpful to respond — "I'm sorry you aren't feeling better — it certainly looks like your strength is better today. You're sitting up by yourself and you were able to eat most of your breakfast." The patient's notion that he is not feeling better is acknowledged but in addition the health professional was able to focus in on the positive signs of improvement that were observable. This intervention helps to short circuit the patient's negative perceptions and gradually aid the patient in realizing that he is getting better.

## CONCLUSION

Allied health and nursing professionals by the very nature of their jobs will encounter people who are not only physically ill but have emotional needs as well. Since physical illness and emotions, usually in the form of anxiety, are so intertwined it is usually not enough to treat just the physical and to ignore the emotional components. As mental health problems can present anywhere, it is important for those health professionals outside of mental health to be able to recognize potential emotional problems that result from physical illness or hospitalization and be comfortable in intervening to lessen the patient's anxiety and distress and possibly enhance his recovery.

In this chapter the focus was upon the use of basic interviewing techniques and skills as a tool in helping to establish a more positive interaction between patients and care providers. Communicating clearly, listening attentively, observing accurately, being empathic were seen as essential skills in attaining a therapeutic and helpful relationship with patients.

## REFERENCES

1. Bingham WV, Moore BV: How to Interview. New York: Harper & Brothers, 1959.

2. Bernstein L, Dana R: Interviewing and the Health Professions. New York: Appleton, Century, Crofts, 1970.

3. Gerrard B, Boniface W, Love B: Interpersonal Skills for Health Professionals. Virginia: Reston Publishing, Co., 1980.

4. Pope B: The Mental Health Interview: Research and Application. New York: Pergamon, 1979.

5. Bernstein L, Bernstein R: Interviewing: A Guide for Health Professionals. New York: Appleton, Century, Crofts, 1980.

6. Leon RL: Psychiatric Interviewing: A Primer. New York: Elsevier, 1982.

7. MacKinnon R, Michels R: The Psychiatric Interview in Clinical Practice. Philadelphia: Saunders, 1971.

8. Johnson W: Basic Interviewing Skills. In: The Clinical Practice of Psychology. Edited by Walker EC. New York: Pergamon Press, 1981.

# Chapter 3

PSYCHODYNAMICS
UNDERSTANDING HIDDEN MEANINGS AND MESSAGES

## RICHARD CARLSON, M.D.

The psychodynamic approach to the understanding of normal and abnormal development of individuals is useful to health and mental health workers because it assists in examining psychological mechanisms. Psychodynamic theory examines the behavior of the person based on his early childhood development and environmental influences. It assumes an ongoing interaction between conscious and unconscious mechanisms, that is, it represents a dynamic or changing psychological process.

## HISTORICAL ROOTS

Sigmund Freud and his daughter Anna Freud are among some of the best known pioneers in the field of dynamic psychiatry. It was postulated by the elder Freud that psychosexual phases through which children passed were major factors in their development (1). These, it was stated, helped shape their future personalities, feelings, behaviors and unconscious mental processes. He felt that these had biological and environmental components, that they were normal developmental phenomena, and disturbances during these milestones would result in psychological symptoms, often so-called neuroses. A neurosis was described as arising from trauma during a psychosexual developmental phase (or phases) and resulted from unconscious mental conflicts. Symptoms of anxiety, phobias, or compulsions are examples of attempts to deal with the conflict.

## PSYCHOSEXUAL DEVELOPMENT

First of all, in psychosexual development, Freud spoke of the "oral phase." This begins at birth, lasts about one year or slightly longer and consists of sucking and biting pleasures of the infant. Intense sensations occur around the mouth during this phase, which may include breast feeding. Intense frustration can also occur in the infant during this period when oral needs are not met. It is also during this time that visual fixations on the nurturing object, usually the mother, and other significant people occur.

During the "anal phase," usually beginning early in the second year and extending into the third year, the child has great interest in and sensation around the activities of anal elimination and its control. This stage is particularly concerned with cleanliness, control, and compliance. It may be seen, then, how important this phase can be on future personality development.

In the "Oedipal (or phallic) phase" the child develops interest in the genitals. This period lasts from about ages three to six. The term "Oedipal" is used to express the growing interest the child has especially towards the parent of the opposite sex. This was derived from the Greek drama *Oedipus Rex*, in which Oedipus kills his father and has an incestuous relationship with his mother. Freud viewed this tale as a central myth of all mankind (2). Freud felt that how the child resolves this problem is important in determining future unconscious conflicts. Usually, the child makes attempts to be more like the parent of the same sex (identification) and realizes that the full attention of the other parent will not be forthcoming. The child then usually becomes interested in play with peers. This phase has much to do with future well-adjusted sexual identity or conflicts in the area of sexuality and assertiveness.

## STRUCTURAL COMPONENTS OF THE PSYCHE

In addition to these dynamic developmental processes in children. Freud is noted for his view of the mind as consisting of functional compartments, namely the ego, id, and superego (3). Although these may have rough neuroanatomical equivalents, they were meant to represent psychologically functioning portions of the brain. Freud systematically described psychic energies and functions as he felt they existed.

The *ego* represents that part of the mind, mostly conscious and aware, which has to do with day-to--day functioning. It deals with logic and reality, mediates between the inner and outer worlds and between the instinctual drives of the id and the prohibitions of the superego. It attempts to keep things in a balance or homeostasis and includes such cognitive processes as thinking, feeling, perception, memory and the so-called ego defense mechanisms.

The *id* consists of unconscious instinctual, sexual and aggressive drives. Unacceptable feelings must be pushed back (repressed) into the id. If they are intense and conflicted, and if the ego cannot successfully ward them off, they may appear as a psychotic process. Otherwise, this conflict may cause intense anxiety in the individual. A so-called neurosis may result if these conflicts are defended against by something such as a compulsion or phobia, for example.

The *superego*, sometimes called the "conscience," represents the moral, right-or-wrong aspect of the mind. Ideals are internalized during development. The child acquires his own internal set of standards based on parental expectations. A too severe superego, in which one could not live up to ideals, may result in harsh self-criticism and can lead to a depression. An adequate superego is essential for functioning in society.


## EGO DEFENSE MECHANISMS

The interactions of these agencies of the mind, conscious (aware) and unconscious (hidden) parts, is really what psychodynamics encompasses. For example, recurring, strong id impulses to physically strike out at authorities may not be conscious in the ego of the person, but what he may be aware of is an inner tension resulting in the feeling of anxiety. As the impulses become stronger and impinge on the ego, the superego (conscience) and ego cannot tolerate them. The person defends against these impulses. In this particular case, the person might have a *conversion* symptom, whereby this impulse energy is converted into a muscle paralysis of the arm, as if the ego were saying to the superego that no violence could  be committed with a useless arm. Another person might employ a defense such as *reaction formation*, in which he would act opposite to his feelings. In this example, the person might  show an over-friendliness and outgoing behavior to authorities. If the person were a schizophrenic with poor ego-functioning and these impulses were to arise, he might use the defense of *projection*, whereby he would automatically assume that others were going to harm him rather than him harming others. This is the basic mechanism of paranoia.

All of these processes just mentioned are called *ego defense mechanisms*. They occur unconsciously and automatically as the ego attempts to fend off anxiety which arises as unconscious id impulses bombard it. Some other ego defenses are the following:

*Repression* — the most common and frequently used. It helps to push back into the unconscious (to "forget") what is not wanted.

*Denial* — disavows external reality which is painful to accept or internal feelings or thoughts which are not wanted.

*Intellectualization* — uses reasoning or thinking processes and cuts off the emotional content.

*Rationalization* — attempts to use reason or logic to explain something and make it acceptable. For example, if a person's spouse left, the person using rationalization would think that the spouse is no-good, and would attempt to justify what happened and not feel sorrow.

*Sublimation* — the transformation of unacceptable impulses, thoughts or feelings into acceptable ones. The person with strong aggressive drives could take up a sport through which these energies could be dissipated and the person likely could be commended on his sporting performance.

*Displacement* — the unacceptable feelings are disguised and placed somewhere else, as in a phobia, where the object of fear is the focus of the displacement.

*Undoing* — the action attempts to undo the unacceptable feelings or impulses, usually resulting in a *compulsion*. Constant cleaning or washing may attempt to undo the desire to soil.

These are some examples of defense mechanisms which occur normally and some which have pathological significance and which appear in symptomatic disorders. Everyone uses some defense mechanisms to maintain an internal equilibrium and a balance with the environment. Some defenses are much more pathological than others, such as denial, displacement and projection, and may lead to further problems by their use. On the other hand, use of them may be representative of a weak ego with poor defense mechanisms, such as in schizophrenia.

## PSYCHODYNAMICS IN DAILY LIFE

We have already seen how some psychodynamic events can express themselves so that they are more visible in the person's feelings, thinking, speech or behavior. We can also see these hidden meanings in daily life. For instance, Freud drew attention to slips of the tongue as being representative of  underlying, unconscious material (4). A man, introducing his wife to someone with: "I would like you to meet my mother Gloria," may have some deep-seated conflicts about women and a strong attachment to his mother. The unconscious is capable of asserting itself sometimes in conscious behavior, and this is a normal phenomenon.

Dreams give us a view of some of our unconscious material. They are disguised, however slightly, by the sleeping ego so they do not usually express themselves in an unadulterated form. The closer they are to the original material, with very little disguise, the more of a nightmare they are. A dream of losing things and not being able to find them the night before a possible job promotion could represent unconscious fears of success and difficulties with competitiveness and aggression.

Children normally are less inhibited when they are quite young and express themselves more blatantly. For instance, a four-year-old boy might say: "Daddy, when you go away next week, can I sleep in your bed with mommy?" Psychotic patients, with poor ego functioning, frequently show unconscious material. A schizophrenic patient might say: "My father is a homosexual and is trying to attack me."

The free-association in psychoanalysis offer some insights into unconscious thoughts and feelings. Hypnosis also attempts to undo repression, so that "forgotten" but stored materials may come into awareness.

## CASE EXAMPLES

Through the understanding of psychodynamics, one can obtain some insights into unconscious thoughts and feelings. This will help in understanding the patient and it will assist the therapist in interpreting events so that they may be clearer to the patient. Furthermore, looking at hidden meanings helps the therapist in assessing the patient and making some assumptions about the past and predictions about possible future behavior. Let us look at some case examples.

> In the first instance, a 25-year-old single female secretary is in psychotherapy because of depression. She has trouble sleeping, loses interest in doing things, doesn't feel like eating and cries at times, but doesn't know why. She has difficulty concentrating and consequently her work is deteriorating. She has moved from job to job and indicates that many of her supervisors were impossible to get along with. She relates the onset of this depression to the arrival of a new supervisor.
>
> She states: "I can't take orders from this woman. She's out to get me fired, I know. She's just like an old lady school teacher who has no feelings. She orders me around and I know she hates me. I'm so depressed when I have to go to work, I wish I could die. I miss work alot and just lay in bed."

In examining this case, it is important to note that this woman is reacting more intensely than would be expected in this type of situation — she has many symptoms and considers dying. Also, the symptoms are continuing and she seeks relief through therapy. She does not want to feel this way. This apparently has also happened in the past, so that some underlying problem needs exploring and resolution.

We must also examine with the patient how realistic the situation is. How difficult is the supervisor? Are others affected? What really is going on? Further assumptions, to be examined later, can be made. She probably has an unconscious conflict with parental-type authority figures. This supervisor may remind her strongly of someone toward whom she had mixed love-hate feelings in the past, such as a parent. She is turning the hate feelings against herself (her superego is reacting) and she is depressed, cries, and thinks of dying. There is a tendency toward regressing to earlier phases of development, because she lies in bed, misses her responsibilities at work, and acts less adult-like. She is projecting some of her aggression in a mildly paranoic way by indicating that the supervisor hates her. She may have had some difficulties during the anal phase of psychosexual development in dealing with authorities (parents). This is evidenced by her recurring difficulties over the years with authorities and her present depression (her harsh superego).

In another case, we are confronted with assessing a 22-year-old single male brought in from his home by the police after threatening to stab his father. His thoughts are disjointed and illogical, he believes that he is a woman that has been transformed into God and he hears voices telling him that he is holy and that others want to crucify him. There is no history of drug abuse. A tentative diagnosis of schizophrenia is made. Further information reveals that the patient has been living with his parents and had a similar episode two years previously, at which time he believed he was Superman and beat up his father.

In assessing this case, we realize that the patient's schizophrenic disorder has relapsed and that he has very poor ego strengths at this time. Unconscious impulses are invading his consciousness. He is attempting to repress them and disguise them, but is barely able to do so. Oedipal conflicts are arising. He wants to kill the father, he does not want to feel less than masculine and believes grandiosely that he is superhuman. He denies his aggression by wanting to be holy and projects his violent feelings outside, thinking others want to harm him.

In treating this man, it should be remembered that his illness could result in violence since he has intense Oedipal conflicts which appear when his ego is weakened. When he is well, these things are repressed into his unconscious.

## SUMMARY

Psychodynamics, and our efforts to observe them, can be helpful in gaining a better understanding of why people do what they do in health and in illness. Sigmund Freud historically set the frame-work for dynamic psychiatry by introducing the concept of infantile sexuality and developmental stages. Studying the functional and structural aspects of the mind further assisted in the understanding of the workings of the psyche. Psychodynamic principles are useful in individual and group psychotherapy (especially Psychoanalytical-type), assessment of patients, understanding child development, as a tool in further research, analysis of symptom formation in psychopathology, and also in observing some of the behaviors of people in everyday life.

## REFERENCES


1. Freud S: Three Essays on the Theory of Sexuality. In: Standard Edition of  the Complete Psychological Works of Sigmund Freud. Vol. 7. London: Hogarth Press, 1905 (b).

2. Freud S: Group Psychology and the Analysis of the Ego. New York: Liveright, 1940.

3. Freud S: The Ego and the Id. In: Standard Edition of the Complete Psychological Works of Sigmund Freud. Vol. 19. London:Hogarth Press, 1923 (a).

4. Freud S: The Psychopathology of Everyday Life. In: Standard Edition of the Complete Psychological Works of Sigmund Freud. Vol. 6. London: Hogarth Press, 1901.

# Chapter 4

COMMUNICATING CROSS-CULTURALLY:<br>
APPRECIATING SOCIO-CULTURAL DIFFERENCES

EDWARD G. SILVERMAN, Ph.D.<br>
EFRAIN A. GOMEZ, M.D.<br>
PEDRO RUIZ, M.D.

The anthropologist Fortune (1) describes a Melanesian culture in which all people were believed to be malevolent and intent on harming one another. In this society, a commonly used polite phrase at the acceptance of a gift was " and if you now poison me, how shall I repay this present?" Indiviudals who periodically created a disturbance by running around trying to stab anyone within their reach with a knife were not seen as abnormal and, in fact, no attmepts were made to control such behavior. Other members of the society kept their distance from such individuals and fled when they saw the attack coming. In contrast, the individual who was consistently regarded as mentally ill was a man who had a sunny, kindly disposition and who liked to share with and be helpful to others. Men and women alike never spoke of this man without laughing and he was considered silly, simple and definitely crazy.

The example cited above certainly indicates that our cultural experience is not an adequate yardstick for judging the behavior of individuals in another culture. The very behavior that is considered abnormal or mentally ill in one society or even in one subculture may be valued and considered admirable in another. And, considering the vast cultural diversity in American society, we need not look beyond our own communities to find significant social differences. Nevertheless, Szasz (2) suggests that when mental health professionals evaluate patients they essentially compare the patient's behavior with their own conceptions of normality, which in turn are influenced by the values of the culture in which they live and work. This may lead to diagnostic errors, stigmatizing labels, inappropriate treatment, and even mental illness induced by self-fulfilling prophecies (3). For these

43

reasons, health and mental health workers must pay very close attention to social–cultural as well as biological and psychological factors when providing care. It is, therefore, important to understand the manner in which cultural background affects the development, presentation and treatment of mental disorders.

## CULTURAL DIFFERENCES IN THE EXPRESSION OF MENTAL DISORDERS

The definition, conception and expression of mental illness differs from culture to culture. For example, Rabkin (4) found significant differences between Western (e.g., American, European) and non-Western (e.g., Asian) public attitudes towards mental illness. Non-western attitudes were characterized by less emphasis on the medical model, more differences between professional and public attitudes, and less willingness to label behavior as deviant. Ruiz (5) emphasizes the importance of this issue when dealing with Hispanic patients. Hispanic patients often perceive mental illness as being caused by "supernatural" phenomenon, whereas mental health professionals trained in the Western hemisphere perceive such illnesses as a "natural" phenomenon. While Western clinicians tend to perceive symptoms in negative terms, Hispanic patients may see certain symptoms as a gift of quality. For example, hallucinatory experiences may be perceived as a sign of mediumship, that is, a special religious quality which could be developed in such a way that the person afflicted with hallucinatory symptoms can be a "healer" in his own right and assist people in need of such healing practices. Although the symptoms may still be an expression of mental illness, a lack of awareness of the patient's understanding of, and attitude towards, these symptoms may lead to a rejection of mental health services or a complete failure in treatment compliance. In addition, there are instances in which the same "symptoms" should not even be considered evidence of mental illness. For example, in large segments of African societies, visions, hallucinations and spirits are shared and accepted as legitimate and normal within the belief system of the culture (6, 7).

Objective mental health evaluations should take into consideration the fact that people with different backgrounds and experiences express distress differently and that the same signs may have different meanings depending upon the cultural context. Even the most common and universal cross-culturally prevalent mental disorders have basic expressive differences among minority cultures. For example, Abad and Boyce (8) reported that Puerto Ricans complained little about depression per se, but rather complained about symptoms of insomnia, eating problems, fatigue, headaches, body aches and feelings of weakness and exhaustion. Similarly, they reported that Puerto Ricans, in general, do not recognize anxiety in and of itself, but instead complain of heart palpitations, dizziness and fainting.

Bintie (9) conducted a study of depression across cultures in an attempt to determine whether depressed individuals in African cultures show typical signs of sin, guilt, and suicidal tendencies. The results indicate that depression in the African cultures studied (Nigeria) is expressed primarily as depressed mood, somatic symptoms and motor retardation. In the European culture studied (Britain), symptoms of depression included guilt, suicidal ideation and anxiety, but less somatic symptoms. Guilt and suicidal ideas or acts were uncommon in African subjects and this suggests that guilt and suicide to a large extent are culturally determined.

The different personal and social environments of Black–Americans also results in differences in the development and presentation of mental illness. In many settings, considerable guardedness and/or hyperalertness is necessary for Black–American survival and so the notion of adaptive paranoia among black patients is an important consideration (10, 11). Black patients can also develop special signs and symptoms of distress. For instance, black patients are more likely to be active and self–destructive in their expressions of depression (12). Activity and agitation are more common and there is a tendency for blacks to express sadness and depression  through anger. In addition, black patients are less likely to cry or lose their appetite when depressed.

Certain culture bound syndromes exist that are neither shared nor even understood by other members of American society or by most representatives of  health care professions. For example, Fernandez-Marina (13) described a unique manifestation among Puerto Ricans which he termed "the Puerto Rican syndrome." This syndrome is characterized by sudden seizure–like activity and is thought to serve to defend against overwhelming aggressive impulses. Although it is important to rule out any neurological or psychiatric disorders which could be masked by this syndrome, it is also important to be aware that such a syndrome is accepted as "normal" within the Puerto Rican culture. Other culture-bound syndromes exist which also imply culture-specific ways of handling conflicts and problems. For example, anthropologists have described Windigo psychosis among the Algonquin Indian hunters in which the starved man is convinced that he is in the power of a supernatural monster with a craving for human flesh (14). Other examples of culture bound syndromes include magical fright of Latin Americans, ghost sickness of the Navajo Indian and voodoo and hoodoo of Black Americans.

Religion is a specific aspect of one's cultural background which strongly influences one's definition of mental health and expression of mental illness. With regard to Hispanic patients, particularly Puerto Ricans, Ruiz (16) has emphasized the importance of understanding the existence of spiritism, witchcraft and black magic and their application to the mental health care system. A good example of this is the fact that although the majority of Puerto Ricans are raised as Catholics, it is estimated that between 31 and 80% of the Puerto Rican population of New York City also practiced spiritism (17). Spiritists attribute various states of ill-health and interpersonal problems to different kinds of spirits which exist in an invisible world. Thus, a clinician whose patient speaks of being in contact with a dead relative, or of having heard the voice of a dead relative, may consider this to be a sign of mental illness without recognizing it as a common and culturally accepted occurrence among Hispanics from the Caribbean area.

Similarly, Glossolalia ("speaking in tongues") is an intense religious experience which has often been explained as a symptom of mental illness. "Speaking in tongues" is one of the distinctive aspects of Pentecostalism which is a rapidly growing religious sect in the United States. Hine (18) reported that Pentecostal individuals in the United States who "speak in tongues" are well-integrated and productive members of society. Explaining an unusual and intense religious experience as a symptom of mental illness when it is a common occurrence in a particular religious group represents a value judgment and a religious bias which may lead to diagnostic errors.

It is well beyond the scope of this chapter to offer a comprehensive overview of each ethnic group with regard to differences in the development and expression of mental illness. The examples cited above only serve to emphasize that such social differences do exist and that cultural beliefs may interweave themselves into the psychiatric evaluation process. Mental health practitioners must be aware that these cultural differences exist and that they commonly manifest themselves in both health and mental health settings.

## THE LANGUAGE BARRIER

Language is another important barrier which must be overcome to achieve effective cross-cultural communication. Language is an important component of any culture or subculture and, in fact, some have even said that culture is language (19). Several studies suggest that the bilingual Hispanic patient appears different when examined in English than when examined in his native Spanish tongue (20). Certainly, much can be lost when the bilingual Hispanic patient thinks in Spanish, translates to himself and then verbalizes in English. Obviously, it would be desirable to employ mental health professionals who both literally and metaphorically "speak the same language" as their patients. Unfortunately, this is often impossible and there is a need for appropriately and adequately trained interpreters. In such cases, it is important to select an interpreter who is familiar with psychiatric terminology, who has a thorough knowledge of the language that is being used, and who has the ability to understand the culture of both the clinician and the patient (21). The interpreter should allow the clinician and the patient to speak to each other as if they were communicating in the same language and should resist the temptation to talk directly with the patient.

Non-verbal communication is as much a part of language and equally as important as verbal fluency. It is important to understand the meaning of gestures, postures and inflections if one is to communicate cross-culturally. These non-verbal messages may harden, soften, emphasize or even contradict what is being communicated verbally. Cross-cultural differences in non-verbal communications are significant. For example, in the main stream Anglo-American culture, direct eye contact typically indicates attention whereas in the Navajo culture, direct stares are considered hostile (22).

Cultural differences in the use of language must also be considered. For example, Anglo-Americans generally view silence adversely; however, in Asian cultures, silence may indicate respect (22). Similarly, some American Indian tribes find silence appropriate for children but for others it is a symptom of withdrawal. Even within certain subcultures of our English speaking society, a language barrier may exist between the clinician who uses standard English and the patient for whom non-standard English is the norm (20). For example, Black-American patients from predominantly lower class backgrounds tend to use shorter sentences and less grammatical elaboration than Anglo patients from middle-class and upper-class backgrounds (22). These differences may lead not only to misunderstanding, but to the erroneous conclusion that blacks are inferior with regard to their intellectual functioning. Similarly, the speech of Appalachian whites tends to be characterized by fewer qualifiers, adjectives and adverbs, especially those which refer to feelings (23). It is essential for the mental health worker to be aware of and not misinterpret these important cultural differences.

In attempting to bridge the language barrier, one must be sensitive in using certain cultural terminology. For example, some people would be offended by the use of the term "Hispanic" throughout this chapter and would prefer to be described as "Latino" or "Chicano." This issue is crucial in trying to ascertain the culture of a patient.

## CULTURAL BARRIERS
## IN CONVENTIONAL TREATMENT

Cultural differences often prevent prospective patients from ever entering the mental health system. Moffic and Adams (24) emphasize that one's cultural background may influence expectations regarding mental health care professionals and the roles played by family members and lay healers. In many cultures and subcultures it is felt that emotional problems are the province of family members and spiritual leaders, certainly not mental health professionals. It has also been reported that families of central European and Eastern backgrounds would rather starve than seek help outside the family for mental problems (25).

Even when patients from so--called minority groups are prompted to seek help from the mental health establishment, they often have trouble relating to the system. Cultural minorities often do not know what is expected of them and may have little knowledge or understanding of the therapeutic process, a culture in and of itself. They typically have little experience with professionals who place the major responsibility for solving one's problems on the patient. Clinicians should structure initial visits (interactions) and let patients know what they intend to do, how they intend to do it and what is expected of them. Extra attention to structuring the clinical situation is necessary when the particular cultural group in question emphasizes a structured and well ordered approach to life (26); this is particularly true for Chinese American families (27). Recent work at the University of Southern California (28) suggests that educating patients about the therapeutic process and clarifying expectations of both patients and therapists may decrease premature terminations and enhance outcome.

In conventional forms of treatment such as psychodynamic psychotherapy, cultural differences have an important impact on the process of therapy and, in particular, on the relationship between the patient and the therapist. Significant differences in racial, ethnic, or socioeconomic backgrounds may seriously hinder the development of rapport. Many cultural minorities teach their children at an extremely early age to be fearful and suspicious of the majority (typically Anglo) culture. For example, Mexican American children in the Southwest fearfully and angrily cry "La migra!" (immigration official) when any official looking vehicle enters the neighborhood (29). Black children learn at an early age that white people are not to be trusted and may continue to have experiences which lead them to approach whites with anxiety, mistrust and resentment. These attitudes certainly make it less likely for patients to disclose their thoughts, feelings and needs to the therapist.

Similarly, attitudes, beliefs, and values of the clinician may have a negative affect on the medical relationship with certain cultural minorities. Difficult as it may be to admit, some clinicians may not like, respect or even accept — let alone understand — some of their patients. Such attitudes may strain the relationship and lead to inappropriate behavior towards the patient. Overt hostility is seldom as much a problem as overly indulgent, overly sympathetic and ingratiating behavior on the part of the clinician.

Black-white psychotherapy relationships have been relatively well-studied and illustrate some of the difficulties that can occur in cross-ethnic interactions (30). Block (31) discusses three kinds of errors that white therapists tend to make when attempting to treat black patients. The first error is "color-blindness" in which the patient is viewed as just another patient and the central importance of color is disregarded. The opposite error is the assumption that all of the black patient's problems can be attributed to a lifetime of oppression which has permanently crippled the personality. This has been termed "the mark of oppression" (32). The third type of therapist error has been described as "the great white father syndrome" (33). This refers to both an authoritarian and condescending attitude in which the white therapist presents himself as an omnipotent figure who means nothing but good for the black patient.

Even when there is a cultural and ethnic "match" between therapist and patient, problems in psychotherapy can occur. Vontress (26) emphasized that minorities are typically so disadvantaged that fellow minorities who are successful are often suspect by other members of their own cultural or ethnic group. The minority achievers may be seen as collaborating with the "enemy" while at the same time precipitating a considerable degree of destructive envy in their minority patients. In other instances of patient-therapist similarity, therapists may identify and empathize too much with their patients to the extent that progress in therapy is handicapped. Interestingly, some studies show that minority patients prefer to be treated by therapists from the dominant culture because they are seen as having more skill, understanding and trustworthiness (34).

Treatment of mental health problems with medication also necessitates attention to cultural factors (24). Many Hispanics, Appalachian whites and other cultural groups who view mental illness as a spell cast by witches, may be unresponsive to drugs. On the other hand, many Curanderos (folk healers) utilize "herbs" and may foster an expectation in their patients that prescription medications will produce instant results (35). Physicians must also be knowledgeable of cross-cultural differences in the metabolism of certain medications. For example, blacks may obtain higher blood levels of certain antidepressant medications resulting in unexpected side effects and treatment failure (36). Traditional medication related procedures may even have unanticipated positive results. For example, a patient who believes primarily in folk medicine may feel that the "blood letting" involved in laboratory blood tests is helpful in exorcising a devil spirit (37).

## TREATMENT ALTERNATIVES

Many of the basic assumptions of mental health treatment reflect a variety of values which are primarily Western or Anglo-American in origin. Such assumptions include the notion that emotional difficulties can produce physical symptoms, that previous events in an individual's life can influence their present behavior, and that talking to a mental health professional can help. An objective, scientific, rational approach to one's problems is typically emphasized and separation–individuation from family members is usually valued as a goal for mature adults. It should be noted, however, that many cultural minorities do not share the assumptions on which Western psychology is based. In many non–Western cultures continued interdependence of family members even as adults is considered ideal and the "leaving home" of adolescence which is so valued in Anglo–American society is considered quite undesirable. There are also many non–Western cultures in which subjective, spiritual and supernatural ways of understanding one's problems are more dominant than a scientific and rational belief system. One obvious example is the common belief among many Hispanics that certain symptoms such as anxiety and insomnia are a result of hexes or bad spirits. It is clear that mental health professionals need to appreciate and accept different values and alternative belief systems if we are going to provide mental health services to a wider cultural variety of patients.

Tailoring treatment approaches to the cultural needs of patients may involve the utilization of other than classical psychiatric treatment approaches. Several people have emphasized the importance of folk healers in providing mental health services to specific minority groups. For instance, Ruiz and Langrod (38) offer an excellent comparison between traditional mental health personnel and native folk healers. Unlike classically trained mental health professionals, folk healers communicate in the same language that their patients use. Rather than trying to treat symptoms believed to be supernatural with natural, scientific approaches, folk healers use methods that are much more closely related to the patient's belief system regarding mental health and mental illness. Folk healers see patients in their own homes, live in the same neighborhood, and understand all the stresses and frustrations that are part of the community in which their patients live. Finally, folk healers do not consider the complete removal of symptoms as a necessary condition for healing the patient. On the contrary, they view the patient's symptoms as a gift or quality and the patient is seen as some one who can control their symptoms by relying on inner strength. Folk healers can certainly serve as cultural consultants to broaden our understanding of relevant cultural and religious phenomena. A close reliance between classically trained mental health workers and folk healers is strongly recommended in the treatment of cultural minorities. The following case report illustrates the importance of this issue.

A 23-year-old Puerto Rican woman was admitted to a psychiatric hospital because of agitation, seizures, and vivid auditory and visual hallucinations. The seizures were characterized by an altered state of consciousness, grinding of teeth, clenching of fists and thrashing of the entire body which usually ended in opisthotonos (a form of spasm in which the head and the heels are bent backwards and the body bowed forward). The hallucinations consisted of visions of her dead mother who presented herself as an angry and deformed woman foaming from the mouth and accusing the patient of unspeakable sexual perversions. The patient's present condition had been precipitated by the patient becoming angry and frustrated with her common-law husband who was reproaching and accusing her of infertility and infidelity. Following her hospitalization, the patient received the diagnosis of atypical psychosis and was treated with neuroleptics and standard psychotherapy, but the condition of the patient worsened. It was then that we responded to a request of the family and a folk healer was called for consultation. The folk healer was able to relate to and understand the plight of the patient. He attributed her unusual behavior to her being possessed by a bad spirit. Since he was a medium, he recommended first the discontinuation of the medication which was making her listless and unresponsive, and second he thought that spiritualist meetings with the patient and the spirit of her dead mother were indicated. In the sessions, the patient confessed with reluctance and shame to homosexual and heterosexual transgressions, following which the patient's behavior changed dramatically. Two weeks later, the patient was discharged from the hospital as fully recovered.

Culturally based alternatives for treating mental illness are as varied and diverse as American society. At the Northeast Mental Health Center in Chinatown, San Francisco, California, the ancient healing art of acupuncture is being used to treat a variety of psychological problems including chronic insomnia, somatic complaints and chronic schizophrenia (39). Acupuncturists believe that a force called "Ch'i" circulates the body along energy paths. They believe that illness can occur if these energy paths are blocked as a result of trauma, poor diet or stress. By inserting needles into certain points on the body, acupuncturists believe that they can restore the natural balance of energy. There are a variety of theories that explain how and why acupuncture works, but Chinese patients probably consider it an accepted means of healing the way most Americans accept the use of medication. By combining the acupuncture program with traditional therapy, the staff at the Northeast Mental Health Center felt that they could attract Chinese people who would normally not seek help for their emotional difficulties from the traditional mental health community.


## CONCLUSIONS AND RECOMMENDATIONS

It is quite clear that the development, presentation and treatment of mental health problems are strongly affected by social and cultural factors. Nevertheless, health and mental health professionals still tend to use their own cultural frame of reference in diagnosing and treating patients. While significant advances in the mental health field have emerged within the last decade in psychological and biological approaches to treatment, relatively little attention has been paid to social and cultural influences. In spite of considerable evidence to the contrary, there is a tendency to assume that patients and mental health specialists share the same values and assumptions regarding mental health and mental illness despite obvious cultural differences. Health and mental health professionals are not typically trained to understand cultural differences and there has been relatively little formal effort to overcome language and cultural barriers in our mental health system.

An attractive but unrealistic solution to the problem would be to make a greater effort to insure that patients and mental health workers are from the same social and cultural background (40). However, proportionately few minority members are trained as mental health workers and this would be difficult considering the number of minority patients. Therefore, health professionals should make every effort to acquire both a knowledge and an understanding of a patient's cultural and social background. The patient should be considered a valuable provider of culturally relevant information. Alternative vlaues and belief systems should be respected and integrated into the treatment program. Anthropologists and sources of information (e.g., folk healers) in the patient's cultural group should be consulted. Health professionals should be open, flexible and willing to modify their treatment approaches to reflect their sensitivity to cultural differences. Finally, we must periodically examine our own values and the attitudes we hold towards our patients.

# REFERENCES


1. Fortune RF: Sorcerers of Dobu. New York: Dutton, 1932.
2. Szasz TS: The Myth of Mental Illness. New York: Harper & Row, 1974.
3. Rosenthal R, Jacobson L: Pygmalion in the Classroom: Teacher Expectation and Pupils' Intellectual Development. New York: Holt, Rinehart and Winston, 1968.
4. Rabkin JG: Public attitudes towards mental illness: a review of the literature. Schizophrenia Bulletin, 10:9-33, 1974.
5. Ruiz P: The Hispanic patient: socio-cultural perspectives, In: Mental Health and Hispanic Americans, Karno M, Escobar JI (Eds). New York: Grune and Stratton, Inc., 1982, pp. 17-27.
6. Draguns JG: Values reflected in psychopathology: the case of the Protestant ethic. Ethos, 2:115-136, 1974.
7. Rin H, Schooler C, Caudill WA: Culture, social structure, and psychopathology in Taiwan and Japan. Journal of Nervous and Mental Disease, 157: 296-213, 1973.
8. Abad V, Boyce G: Issues in psychiatric evaluations of Puerto Ricans: a socio-cultural perspective. Journal of Operational Psychiatry, 8(2):52-63, 1977.
9. Binitie A: A factor-analytic study of depression across cultures (African and European). British Journal of Psychiatry, 127:559-563, 1975.
10. Grier WH, Cobbs PM: Black Rage. New York: Basic Books, 1968.
11. Griffith MS, Jones EE: Race and psychotherapy: changing perspectives. Current Psychiatric Therapies, 18:225-235, 1979.
12. Poussaint AF: Why Blacks Kill Blacks. New York: Emerson Hall, 1972.

13. Fernandez-Marina R: The Puerto Rican Syndrome: its dynamics and cultural determinants. Psychiatry, 24:79-82, 1961.

14. Ullman P, Krasner L: A Psychological Approach to Abnormal Behavior. Englewood Cliffs, NJ: Prentice-Hall, Inc., 1969.

15. Kiev A: Transcultural Psychiatry. New York: Free Press, 1972.

16. Ruiz P: Spiritism, mental health and the Puerto Ricans: an overview. Transcultural Psychiatric Research, Vol. XVI:28-43, 1979.

17. Garrison V: The Puerto Rican Syndrome in psychiatry and spiritism, In: Case Studies in Spirit Possession, Crapanzano V, Garrison V (Eds). New York: John Wiley & Sons, Inc., 1977, pp. 383-449.

18. Hine VH: Pentecostal glossolalia — toward a functional interpretation. Journal for the Scientific Study of Religion, 8:211-226, 1969.

19. Martinez C Jr.: Hispanics: Psychiatric Issues. Paper presented at Symposium on Current Psychiatric Diagnosis and Treatment Issues in Blacks and Hispanics. Houston, Texas: June, 1982.

20. Ruiz P, Silverman EG: Emergency psychiatric services to minorities, In: Phenomenology and Treatment of Psychiatric Emergencies, Comstock BS, Fann WE, Pokorny AD, Williams RL (Eds). Jamaica, NY: Spectrum Publications, Inc., (in press).

21. Cox JL: Psychiatric assessment of the immigrant patient. British Journal of Hospital Medicine, 16:38-40, 1976.

22. Sue DW, Sue D: Barriers to effective cross-cultural counseling. Journal of Counseling Psychology, 24:420-429, 1977.

23. Weller JE: Yesterday's People: Life in Contemporary Appalachia. Lexington, KY: University of Kentucky Press, 1966.

24. Moffic HS, Adams GL: Sociodemographic influences on evaluation and treatment, In: A Clinician's Manual on Mental Health Care: A Multidisciplinary Approach. Moffic HS, Adams GL (Eds). Menlo Park, CA: Addison-Wesley, 1982, pp. 205-217.

25. Giordino J, Giordino GP: Ethnicity and community mental health. Community Mental Health Review, 1:1-26, 1976.

26. Vontress CE: Racial and ethnic barriers in counseling, In: Counseling Across Cultures, Pedersen PP, Draguns JG, Lonner WJ, Trimble JE (Eds). The University of Hawaii Press, 1981, pp. 87-107.

27. Sue DW, Sue S: Counseling Chinese-Americans. Personnel and Guidance Journal, 50:637-644, 1972.

28. Fields S: Telling it like it is. Innovations, 6(2):3-7, 1979.

29. Moore JW: Mexican Americans. Englewood Cliffs, NJ: Prentice-Hall, Inc., 1970.

30. Griffith M: The influence of race on the psychotherapeutic relationship. Psychiatry, 40:27-32, 1977.

31. Block CB: Black Americans and the cross-cultural counseling and psychotherapy experience, In: Cross-Cultural Counseling and Psychotherapy, Marsella AJ, Pedersen PB (Eds). New York: Pergamon Press, 1981, pp. 177-194.

32. Kardiner A, Ovesey L: The Mark of Oppression. New York: Norton, 1951.

33. Vontress CE: Counseling Negroes. New York: Houghton-Mifflin, 1971.

34. Fields S: Mental health and the melting pot. Innovations, 6(2):2, 1979.

35. Snow L: Folk medical beliefs and their implications for care of patients. Annals of Internal Medicine, 81:82-96, 1974.

36. Ziegler V, Briggs J: Tricyclic plasma levels. Journal of American Medical Association, 238:2167-2169, 1977.

38. Ruiz P, Langrod J: The role of folk healers in community mental health services. Community Mental Health Journal, 12:392-398, 1976.

39. Fields S: Ancient needles for modern ills. Innovations, 6(2):14-15, 1979.

40. Shapiro ET, Pinsker H: Shared ethnic scotoma. American Journal of Psychiatry, 130:1338-1341, 1973.

# Chapter 5

GENERAL ETHICAL AND THERAPEUTIC PRINCIPLES:
DO NO HARM

BRUCE MARCH, M.A.
RANJIT C. CHACKO, M.D.

Along with recent advances in medical science, there have been accompanying ethical problems. The popular literature has reported many ethical dilemmas which now exist in medical science. Ethical issues concerning abortion, organ transplantation, brain death and passive euthanasia are all receiving media attention.

It is apparent that we are living in an age of accountability. Those making decisions and performing actions which affect the welfare of others are expected to be competent performers as well as cognizant of the rights of their charges. Recent court cases in the political and medical arenas have illustrated current concerns with accountability.

The mental health care professions have also been affected by this "age of accountability." Although lacking the media attention focused on non–psychiatric medicine and politics, there is growing social and legal pressure to compel helping professionals to be more accountable for their actions.

Every helping professional could benefit from an understanding of ethics. "What not to do" can be as important as "what to do." Unfortunately, many curriculum programs underemphasize the former. A knowledge and understanding of basic mental health ethics can increase ones effectiveness as a clinician as well as protect one's self and/or agency from law suit.

An examination of professional ethics requires a definition of ethics as well as some brief historical background. In addition, several major issues concerning clinical care will be discussed. The health provider who learns and develops effective therapeutic skills can potentiate much change in their patients. However, it is the understanding and application of ethics which helps the counselors' interventions "to do no harm."

## WHAT ARE ETHICS?

The term ethics derives from the Greek word ethos which means custom or character. In the context of current usage, ethics can be defined as "the principle of conduct governing an individual or a group" (1).

Most professional organizations of mental health service providers have established codes of ethics to provide guidelines for their members. For example, the American Nurses Association (2), American Psychological Association (3), American Psychiatric Association (4), and the National Association of Social Workers (5) have all developed and published their own ethical standards. It is important that one be aware of the ethical guidelines for one's own professional area. However, the guidelines of these organizations tend to be minimal standards and by no means cover every situation. In fact, occasionally two ethical standards applied to the same situation may demand opposing modes of action, resulting in an "ethical dilemma."

When faced with an ethical dilemma, or a difficult question concerning interpretation of ethical standards, one tends to be greatly influenced by personal values. In fact, personal values of the clinician can have great impact on clinical care. One area of clinical care where these values are particularly evident is in the psychotherapeutic or counseling process.

## ROLE OF VALUES IN THE CLINICAL PROCESS

A personal value is an individual's belief about the importance, worth or merit of an idea as measurable on a continuum ranging from positive to negative. For example, laziness tends to have a negative social value and ambitiousness tends to have a positive social value.

A therapist's personal values flavors his interpretation of ethical counseling procedures and also has influence on the therapeutic goal setting and techniques of interventions. Some counselors are "value persuaders" and they believe that it is their task to persuade patients to adopt the therapists own personal values. For example, a counselor may believe that a patient's dysfunctional marriage is preferable over the stigma of divorce, and strongly advises the client to remain married. If the patient has given considerable thought to the decision of divorce and has realistic expectations about its consequences, is the counselor overstepping his ethical boundaries?

Other therapists can be described as "value hiders." These counselors strive to be secretive about their values for fear they may influence their patient's decisions. For example, a patient states he intends to earn a living by panhandling, despite the fact he has the ability to hold a regular job. The patient asks the therapist for his opinion but the therapist avoids responding. Is a value free stance conducive to effective psychotherapy?

"Value hiders" and "value persuaders" do not make effective therapists. "Value hiders" are seldom successful in keeping their values hidden and provide poor reality testing for their patients. "Value persuaders" tend to act as agents of social conformity and foster much resistance or dependency from their patients.

A clinician's values will emerge in therapy or other clinical interactions. Menninger (6) states that "what a psychoanalyst believes, what he lives for, what he loves, what he considers to be good and what he considers to be evil, become known to the patient and influence him enormously." The question remains as to how to deal with personal values as they arise in the context of providing allied health services. First, it is important for clinicians to be aware of their values as they arise in the course of clinical interactions. Second, clinicians must monitor the impact of their values on treatment and be able to recognize and counteract any situation when treatment becomes indoctrination. Finally, allied health professionals must be prepared to have their values questioned by their patients. Oftentimes such questioning is a form of reality testing — the patient wants to know if his perception of circumstances are congruent with the perception of others. Values often become important focal points of mental health care.

Values are the foundation of our ethical and legal systems. Helping professionals continue to seek concrete norms by which they can guide their therapeutic interventions. Why are ethical codes being sought? First, the development of ethical codes for helping professionals was prompted by a concern for the welfare of mental health consumers. A second factor in the development of ethical principles has been the influence of the judicial system. A code of ethics provide the court a standard by which to judge mental health professionals who are accused of negligence or malpractice. Therefore, a clinician can use a code of ethics as guidance and justification for therapeutic action. Drane (7) points out that providing competent psychotherapy is not necessarily the same as providing ethical psychotheapy. In other words, having clinical skill and knowledge is not sufficient in providing ethical mental health services.

## HISTORICAL BACKGROUND

The study of ethics and ethical problems has occurred for thousands of years. Most religions provide a code of ethical standards. The ten commandments serve this role for Jews and Christians. Ancient Greek philosophers such as Socrates, Plato and Aristotle addressed ethical issues (8).

The role of ethics in the provision of psychotherapy to the mentally ill has become a major concern only recently. In the middle ages, the mentally ill were imprisoned and tortured with little regard to their personal rights. The philosophy of English common law, from which most of our laws today are derived, was that the King of England had the authority to act as the guardian of the mentally ill. This guardianship role is known as "parens patriae" and it was accompanied by police power which enabled the state to remove mentally ill people from society when they represented a threat to the welfare of other citizens.

In the middle of the nineteenth century, there was a movement in the United States to create state mental hospitals which would provide treatment for the mentally ill. Until that time there were few hospitals and many mentally ill people were warehoused in prisons. There were few statutes concerning admission policies and often hospital administrators would make the ultimate decision concerning admission, based on their own perception of dangerousness.

The efforts of activists such as Dorothea Dix brought about reforms concerning the admission process. A new development was statutes providing the right of a jury trial before a patient could be involuntarily committed to a mental hospital. An accompanying change was that many states allowed for commitment based on symptoms of mental illness other than dangerousness.

The principles of "parens patriae" and "police power" still form a basis for current commitment laws. However, these principles apply only to those involuntarily committed, and statutes have been refined to limit the extent to which patient rights can be violated. It is important to realize that the fact that a person is admitted to a mental hospital does not imply that the person is incompetent and surrenders his civil rights. He does not lose the right to make decisions for himself when admitted unless he is found incompetent and a guardian is appointed. This has received much court attention over the last two decades.

The judicial system has recently been very active in outlining the rights of the mentally ill. Many of the courts' decisions involve the protection of rights of hospitalized patients. However, the courts have also addressed specific ethical issues which concern the rights of out-patients who receive counseling. The courts' decision in malpractice and negligence cases against therapists sheds light on standards expected for ethical clinical practice.

## LEGAL RIGHTS OF THE MENTALLY ILL

The American Judicial System has become increasingly concerned about the legal rights of mental health patients. For example, the courts have ruled that when mentally ill patients are committed to a psychiatric hospital they have a right to receive adequate treatment. The case involved a class action suit by a large group of psychiatric patients who were involuntarily hospitalized in Alabama state hospitals. The facilities were found to be below the minimum level at which adequate treatment could occur. The court ruled that treatment must be provided. Treatment was expected to be humane, executed by sufficient and qualified staff and that each patient was entitled to an individual treatment plan.

Another case involving the issue of right to treatment is O'Connor vs. Donaldson (10). This case reached the U.S. Supreme Court. Donaldson was committed to a state mental hospital and kept there for 15 years despite his attempts to seek release on the grounds that he was not dangerous or mentally ill, and that the hospital did not provide him with any treatment. Donaldson's suit contended that the defendent had "intentionally and maliciously deprived him of his constitutional right to liberty." Testimony revealed that Donaldson represented no danger prior to, or during his hospital stay. The Supreme Court ruled in favor of Donaldson stating that his confinement was a "simple regime of enforced custodial care, not a program designed to alleviate or cure his supposed illness." This case is interpreted as stipulating that hospitals cannot confine without treatment a non–dangerous person who is capable of surviving safely in the community.

A second issue which is receiving increasing judicial attention is the right of psychiatric patients to refuse treatment, even when involuntarily committed. A patient involuntarily committed is often not ruled incompetent, so he may refuse treatment. This predicament creates an ethical dilemma. Helping professionals are expected to provide appropriate treatment to the mentally ill but the mentally ill have the right to receive information about proposed treatment and then consent to, or refuse such treatment. Most litigation concerning refusal of involuntary treatment concerns obtrusive therapies such as electroconvulsive shock therapy (ECT) and psychosurgery. Recently, the right of mentally ill patients to refuse psychotropic drugs has reached the courts (11). Certain drugs known as neuroleptics have been found to be very effective anti-psychotic agents and have done much to help many psychiatric patients to return to the community rather than spend long periods of time in the hospital. These medications may present troublesome side-effects such as muscle stiffness, cramping or tremors, and drowsiness. Many of these side-effects can be managed with medication adjustments or additional medication. However, one side effect, a neurological syndrome called tardive dyskinesia, is often not reversible. Prolonged medication use can result in uncontrollable body movements, including tremors of the tongue and contortions of the trunk or extremities.

A case currently before the United States Supreme Court, Mill vs. Rogers (11) argues that the side-effects induced by medication violates patients' constitutional rights. A Federal District Court ruled that except in emergencies, mental patients who are legally competent have an absolute right to refuse treatment with anti-psychotic medication. The judge stated, quoting late Associate Justice Cardozo, that "every human being of adult years and sound mind has a right to determine what shall be done with his own body."

Another issue addressed by the courts concerns a concept known as the "least restrictive alternative." Courts tend to support the principle that in treating a psychiatric patient, the patient has the right to be treated in the least restrictive environment. For example, a patient should not be compelled to be placed in a locked ward when he can receive sufficient therapy on an out-patient basis. Some states have statutes which are intended to enforce this principle. It is essential to note that a psychiatric patient's needs change over time, so frequent re-evaluation is needed to ensure the patient remains in the appropriate level of restrictive environment.

## A QUESTION OF ETHICS?

Medical and mental health caregivers often find themselves in clinical interactions which require difficult ethical decisions. The following case represents the ethical issue of confidentiality.

> A 24-year-old unmarried schizophrenic woman is being seen at an out-patient medical clinic. She informs the medical allied health professional that she has been sexually active with a male friend but neither uses contraceptives. The caregiver refers the patient to a family planning center but the patient refuses to use contraceptives because it is a "hassle." The allied health worker, worried about her patient becoming pregnant, informs the patient's mother. Is this a violation of the patient's right to confidentiality?

Practitioners of health and mental health care have a professional obligation to maintain confidentiality of their relationship with their patients. Most patients expect that the content of their clinical interactions, psychiatric records, medical reports as well as correspondence will remain confidential to treatment team members; and without such expectancy, the process of clinical care will be hindered.

Confidentiality is not an absolute right in all situations. There are times when it is in the best interest of the patient to violate confidentiality. The circumstances by which confidentiality can be violated are not clearly presented by professional ethical standards or judicial decisions. Clinicians often must exercise their own professional judgment in deciding when it is appropriate to reveal information about their patients.

There is general professional agreement that confidentiality should only be broken when not to do so would present a clear danger to the patient or to others. If one is providing services to a depressed patient who reveals that he has decided to end his life, and the clinician has reason to believe the client represents a clear danger to himself, the clinician is expected to intervene. Betraying the patient's trust and warning family members so that they may take precautions, or enlisting the aid of others to facilitate hospitalization would be appropriate action. Those who take large risks in providing services to suicidal clients may find themselves at risk for legal action or negligence (12).

It is also expected that confidentiality will be broken when patients represent a potential danger to others. The case of Tarasoff vs. the Regents of the University of California (13) did much to foster consideration of this issue. A male student receiving therapy from the University counseling center threatened to kill a young woman friend. He had made these threats during therapy sessions and the therapist believed there was enough risk to contact campus police and request they take him into custody until he could be placed in a hospital for observation. However, the police interviewed the man and decided he was not dangerous and released him advising him to stay away from the young woman. For the next two months the woman was out of the country but upon return she was murdered by the patient. The woman's parents sued the therapist, the university, and campus police for not warning the victim of danger, and won the case. The California Supreme Court's final decision stated the therapist's responsibility might "call for him to warn the intended victim or others likely to apprise the victim of the danger, to notify the police or to take whatever steps reasonably necessary under the circumstances."

Occasionally, mental health workers are asked to testify in court cases involving their patients. Gumper and Sprenkle (14) point out that many helping professionals have a false sense of security in believing they are protected by the legal concept of "privileged communication." In reality, statutes in the different states are far from uniform in describing what professional disciplines are covered by this privilege. Although most states give legal privilege to psychiatrists and more recently psychologists, other helping professionals are seldom protected. Another important distinction concerning legal privilege must be made. Privileged communication belongs to the client and not to the therapist. It is the client who may decide to evoke the principle, and not the therapist. With authorization from the client to disclose information, the therapist cannot claim legal privilege.

It is often helpful to advise patients at the onset of contact of their limits to confidentiality. Such discussion creates realistic expectations and avoids creating crises concerning confidentiality in later phases of therapy.

In certain situations, health and mental health workers may be acting as agents for parties other than their clients. For example, an allied health worker may be interviewing prisoners for the legal justice system. In such instances, patients should be advised of how interview information will be utilized.

Patients will often consent to waive confidentiality. A depressed patient may want his therapist to explain the disorder to his family. Another patient may agree to have his sessions videotaped to be employed as a training tool for nursing students. It is important that patients provide written consent when waiving confidentiality. It is also essential that the consent form specifically describe the type of breach of information being allowed.

Ethical questions also arise concerning the issue of informed consent. Patients receiving treatment should be given an option, based on relevant knowledge, to refuse or accept that particular treatment. The type and amount of information and the number of treatment options provided all are integral components of ethical practice. The following case illustrates the ethical concept of informed consent.

> A patient comes to a community mental health clinic with affective complaints and a history consistent with Bipolar Disorder (Manic Depression). The patient, currently in remission, has never been hospitalized or on psychotropic medication. The interviewing psychiatrist and all of the intake staff agree that the patient is manic depressive and would likely benefit from medication, specifically, lithium carbonate. The psychiatrist informs the patient that his psychiatric problems would likely be alleviated if he were to take lithium. The patient, reluctant to take medication, questions the doctor about the nature of his illness and possible drug side-effects. The physician responds that there is little time available to respond to such questions and that the information he desires is quite complex and beyond a layman's understanding. The patient responds by hesitantly agreeing to take the medication. Consent was obtained in this case, but was it "informed consent"?

People receiving mental health services are assumed to be competent unless found otherwise in a court hearing. Therefore, mental health patients have a right to refuse any kind of treatment. They also must consent to treatment they receive and be provided enough information about proposed treatment and alternate treatments available so that they can make an informed choice. In this case of the newly diagnosed manic depressive, there is certain information the patient is entitled to receive. He can make an informed choice only after receiving a basic understanding of his illness, and potential treatments and their respective benefits and shortcomings.

Sometimes a patient chooses a treatment method that is viewed as less effective than the treatment team's choice. However, treatment staff must continue to provide support and services which meet professional standards. Davis (15) points out that informed consent must also be obtained before psychiatric patients can be research participants. Research subjects should be volunteers and be aware that they can discontinue participation at any time. All unnecessary risks should be eliminated and patients should be aware of any remaining risks. Informed consent should be obtained in writing from both research and treatment patients.

Clinicians are expected to practice within the area of their own professional competence. Specifying one's own area of competence requires sound ethical judgment. The following case example illustrates a situation requiring such judgment.

> A patient is referred to a dietician to help him manage his newly diagnosed diabetes. After a few sessions it becomes clear that the patient is an amphetamine abuser. Although the health care provider lacks extensive knowledge or experience in treating drug abusers, he decides to attempt to assist the man discontinue drugs in conjunction with the nutritional counseling. Is this an ethical decision?

It is important that health and mental health professionals recognize their own limitations. Dieticians should not be treating drug problems any more than nurses should be administering psychological tests or social workers should be giving information to clients about the results of laboratory testing. How does one determine his own area of competence? The area of study in which one's degree is earned, the level of that degree, as well as licensure and certifications held are important considerations in assessing one's competence areas. However, most degrees and certifications tend to be generic. For instance, a psychologist may be competent in working in a school setting, yet not be competent in working in an in-patient psychiatric ward. Each health and mental health professional must critically analyze his own clinical skills and knowledge to determine his own competence area. At the same time, each clinician must analyze his clinical deficits and not be afraid to recognize his limitations.

When a clinician encounters a case he cannot provide competent care to, it is important to make an appropriate referral. To make an effective referrral, one must be aware of available psychological and social services as well as clinical specialists in the community. It is also important to recognize when working with a patient who is not making progress, that a consultation is indicated. In such a case, the clinician should enlist the help of a person skilled in the problem area to obtain treatment recommendations, which may, at times, include referring the client elsewhere.

Competent mental health workers will not remain competent unless they continue to pursue knowledge and additional therapeutic skills. The American Nursing Association and many other professional organizations recognize the need for continuing education and professional development, and support efforts to make continuing education a prerequisite for renewal of licensure or certification.

Ethical clinical care includes the documentation of treatment provided to patients as well as patients' response to treatment. The following case reflects the importance of competent documentation.

> During group therapy, a patient on a locked inpatient psychiatric ward discloses to a nurse that he has recently developed strong self-destructive impulses. The nurse fails to note the patient's statement in his chart. That same day, after reviewing the patient's record and finding no contraindications, the patient's therapist grants him a weekend pass. The patient attempts suicide over the weekend.

The above example presents an extreme but convincing argument for accurate documentation in clients' psychiatric records. The written representations of clients' problems, treatment plans, and progress reports are all much needed safeguards for patients and therapists alike. Documentation in patients' charts is a method of sharing information with other treatment personnel, as well as a monitoring device of a patient's progress. Documentation may also protect mental health professionals from legal action. An accurate description of a patient's behavior or condition can justify one's treatment approach. In addition, documentation is evidence that the patient's needs are being met by treatment staff. Notes in a patient's record should be descriptive but brief enough so that they will be read. All crisis episodes and the resulting intervention should be recorded. Entries in a client's record may at some time be available to the patient or others, so entries must be acceptable to such scrutiny.

## OBSTACLES TO PROVIDING EFFECTIVE TREATMENT

Health and mental health workers enter their profession for numerous reasons. A reason commonly cited is "I like to help others." Such altruism can in itself be very rewarding. However, some helping professionals may also use their therapeutic relationships to meet certain inappropriate personal needs. Some clinicians may consciously or unconsciously create therapeutic situations by which their patients become overly dependent on, or idolizing of, the clinician. Rather than teach problem solving to the patient, the clinician seeks to meet his own needs for admiration by, or control of others. Personal needs of the clinician, thereby become obstacles to effective treatment.

Some clinicians use patient contact to meet their own needs for personal problem solving. These clinicians spend much time self–disclosing about their own personal problems and personal triumphs. For example, a physical therapy technician may spend most of his session with a paraplegic talking about his own financial problems. Some self-disclosure may be helpful in developing a therapeutic relationship but caution is advised. By excessive self-disclosure the technician is revealing a narcissistic unwillingness to concentrate on the client's problems.

Some clinicians become over–involved with patients. Such clinicians may enter into social relationships with their patients, while some become romantically involved. Social involvement with patients is certainly non–therapeutic and should be avoided. Sexual contact with patients can, and often does, lead to malpractice suits as well as loss of certification or licensure to conduct treatment.

Caplan (16) points out that beginning clinicians may at times lose their objectivity and as a result become too close to, or distant from a patient to provide effective treatment. Caplan cites some of the causes of this loss of objectivity, and among them are: direct personal involvement, simple identification, and transference. Direct personal involvement includes situations such as the clinician entering into a social relationship with a patient. Simple identification occurs when the clinician identifies with rather than empathizes with the patient or another actor in the clinical picture. For example, a married male clinician may be seeing a couple in marital sessions. The wife may admit to an extramarital affair. The clinician may identify with the hurt and anger experienced by the husband and the clinician may begin to take a punitive and aggressive stance in his interaction with the wife in therapy.

A third cause of lack of objectivity is countertransference. Some clinicians unconsciously distort their relationships to their clients. The clinician may transfer feelings and attitudes toward key figures in the past onto current patients. This transference leads to pre–determined attitudes and expectations on the part of the therapist onto the patients or a significant person in the patient's life. For example, a young female allied health professional grew up in a home with an alcoholic father who eventually abandoned the family. The health care provider held much unresolved anger toward her father. This clinician had a very difficult time treating patients with alcohol abuse problems. She tended to try to instill guilt for their drinking and irresponsible behavior rather than seek causes for their drinking or explore treatment options.

It is apparent from the preceding discussion that personal needs of clinicians can interfere with the provision of effective treatment. An additional obstacle to effective treatment concerns the demands that health and mental health systems impose on clinicians. All clinicians work within a system which makes demands concerning attitudes and behavior of the clinician. Helping professionals working within large institutional settings, such as mental health clinics, hospitals or schools face complex system demands. Clinicians are expected to protect the welfare of their agencies as well as their patients. Clinicians often are overworked, and have few resources available to help patients. There are times when some care providers suffer from "burnout syndrome." This occurs when clinicians become fatigued and pessimistic about their impact in assisting patients. They ask "is all my effort worthwhile?" There are a few methods available to reduce the chances of, or severity of, clinician burnout. First, open discussion about job pressures and frustrations between health or mental health workers and their supervisors can alleviate tension. Second, clinicians who have other rewarding professional and outside activities are more immune to clinician burnout.

Clinicians in multi-service provider settings must support each other's role in providing health and mental health services. The team treatment approach cannot be effective when clinicians conspire with patients to keep secrets from other staff members or share critical comments about other staff members. The result of sharing staff problems with patients is counterproductive to effective treatment. Such action tends to demoralize patients by causing poor confidence in the staff's ability to work together in solving patient problems. When problems develop between staff members concerning treatment methods or personal issues, the appropriate place for discussion is with a supervisor.

Mental health workers must be relatively free of distractions in order to provide effective treatment. A clinician under the influence of alcohol or other illicit drug cannot make clear and effective clinical decisions. In addition, a clinician with a severe personal problem may be too distracted to provide adequate treatment. Clinicians with severe personal problems should be receiving treatment or, like an intoxicated clinician, should remain away from the clinical setting until the problem has passed. Consultation with one's supervisor may be helpful in determining when one's personal problems may have damaging effects on providing clinical care.

## CONCLUSION

During this age of accountability, there has been an increasing amount of attention paid to patients' rights. Some hospitals have hired advocates to represent patients who believe their rights have been violated. The American Hospital Association (17) has issued a patient's Bill of Rights which includes such areas as informed consent, right to refuse treatment and confidentiality.

Health and mental health workers must be aware of the role ethics plays in their every day interaction with patients. They must not be afraid to apply ethical analysis to their decisions or consult with a supervisor when faced with an ethical dilemma.

In addition, health professionals must familiarize themselves with state law and current court trends. What mental health specialties are covered by privileged communication in your state? Can a patient on an out-patient commitment be compelled to take medication? What are licensure laws for psychologists in your state? Such information is most readily accessible in the form of workshops or in-services from experts in mental health law.

It is essential that health and mental health workers and their professional organizations address the issues of ethics and mental health care. If health and mental health professionals do not take the initiative in creating and advocating ethical standards, the responsibility will be assumed by others who may lack the knowledge or understanding of mental health services to adequately complete the task.

Providers of mental health services must be aware of their own values as well as the impact of these values on their patients. Caution must also be taken that clinicians do not lose sight of the patient/care-giver relationship and bring their own issues into the clinical intervention. A health or mental health professional who is cognizant of ethical, legal and clinical principles is better prepared to "do no harm."

## REFERENCES


1. Woolf H (Ed.): Webster New Collegiate Dicitonary. Springfield: G & C Merriam, 1979.

2. American Nurses Association: Guidelines for Implementing the Code for Nurses. Kansas City: The Association, 1980.

3. American Psychological Association: Ethical Principles of Psychologists (1981 Revision). Washington, DC, 1981.

4. American Medical Association: Principles of Medical Ethics with Annotations Approved by the American Psychiatric Association, 1978.

5. National Association of Social Workers: Code of Ethics of the National Association of Social Workers. Washington, DC, 1980.

6. Menninger K: Theory of Psychoanalytic Technique. New York: Basic Books, 1958.

7.  Drane J: Ethics and Psychotherapy: A Philosophical Perspective. In: Ethics and Values in Psychotherapy, Rosenbaum M (Ed.). New York: The Free Press, 1982.

8.  Rosenbaum M: The Issue of Ethics. In: Psychotherapy, Rosenbaum M (Ed.). New York: The Free Press, 1983.

9.  Wyatt vs. Stickney, 344 F Supp. 373, 1972.

10.  O'Connor vs. Donaldson, 422, U.S. 563, 1975.

11.  Applebaum P: Can Mental Patients Say No to Drugs? New York Times Magazine, 46, March 21, 1983.

12.  Perr D: Legal Aspects of Suicide. In: Suicide: Theory and Clinical Aspects, Henhoff D and Ernsidler B (Eds.). Massachusetts: PSG Publishing, 1979.

13.  Tarasoff V: Regents of the University of California, California Reports, 3rd Series, 425.

14.  Gumper L and Sprenkel D: Privileged Communications in Therapy: Special Problems for the Family and Couples Therapist. Family Process, 20:11, 1981.

15.  Davis A: Legal and Ethical Issues. In: Comprehensive Psychiatric Nursing, Haber J, Yeach A, Schudy S and Sidelau B (Eds.). New York: McGraw Hill, 1982.

16.  Caplan G: The Theory and Practice of Mental Health Consultation. New York: Basic Books, 1970.

17.  Countryman K: Development and implementation of a patient's Bill of Rights in hospitals. Chicago: American Hospital Association, 1980.

# Chapter 6

PSYCHIATRIC DIAGNOSIS:
DETERMINING WHAT IS WRONG

PEDRO RUIZ, M.D.
PEDRO P. RUIZ

The field of mental health has reached a high level of sophistication in recent years, particularly with the introduction of the Third Edition of the Diagnostic and Statistical Manual of Mental Disorders in 1980 (1). With the advent of this manual, known as the DSM-III, appropriate recognition has been given to the concern, which has existed for about a decade, of establishing appropriate diagnosis in all mental cases, in such a way that most clinicians, as well as research investigators, could commonly understand and communicate about it. No one in the mental health field will dispute the fact that all quality-oriented treatment programs must begin with an accurate clinical evaluation and diagnostic criteria. Differential diagnosis and appropriate follow-up evaluation can only be made possible if the clinicians in question possess all of the clinical skills and assessment tools needed for the establishment of an accurate diagnosis. This concept has been so well recognized in the field that a training manual has been recently published (2), and is now widely used in most educational institutions in this country dedicated to the training of mental health practitioners. Along these lines, a series of publications (3, 4, 5, 6) have recently focused on the appropriate utilization of the Third Edition of the Diagnostic and Statistical Manual of Mental Disorders, as well as on its most beneficial aspects to the field and some of its disadvantages as well. Of course, every scientist in the field will undoubtedly accept the fact that there are so far no clear-cut definitions that delineate the boundaries of the concept of mental disorders or mental illness. However, it behooves all of us to accept the necessary criteria which will assist in structuring our clinical data in such a way that one could reasonably postulate, in an integrated manner, all of the biological, social, and psychological dysfunctions observed in the clinical situations confronted by mental health practitioners in their day-to-day professional practice. It is within this framework that this chapter is written. Hopefully, the material discussed here will assist the mental health practitioners in becoming better clinicians and diagnosticians, and therefore better able to help their patients with their problems and suffering.

## DATA BASE IN PSYCHIATRY AND THE PRINCIPLES OF THE MENTAL STATUS EXAMINATION

In this section, I would like to address those areas in which most mental health practitioners base their judgments when trying to establish a diagnosis and/or when designing a treatment plan for a given patient. These sources of information constitute what is known as the data base, and in particular, within the data base, the mental status examination. They are as follows:

### Identifying Information

This is the name, age, address, occupational status, marital status, family constellation  and referral sources on a given patient. All these informational resources will skillfully be used by the clinicians in trying to understand the background of the patient, as well as relevant issues that could bring light in exploring, later on, the biological, psychological and social pictures in the case in question.

### Chief Complaint

When trying to elucidate the patient's chief complaint, the clinicians gain insight into what has motivated the patient to secure emotional help, and in many cases, what has motivated the patient's relatives and/or friends to take initiatives along these lines on the patient's behalf. Of course, what constitutes a chief complaint does not, in many cases, constitute the core of the conflict, and therefore, the clinician must know how to apply judgment in this regard when the case requires such a discrimination.

## History of Present Illness

Securing this information will offer the diagnosticians abundant information, all of which is relevant in understanding the process of the illness being dealt with. For instance, the duration of the symptomatology, the time and mode of onset of the illness, the gravity and severity of the problems being confronted, as well as other important clues, will permit the evaluator to integrate all of the information secured in a manner that makes sense from a clinical point of view.

## Childhood History

By securing this information, the evaluator will be able to focus on early patterns of abnormal behavior, early traumatic experiences, and childhood illnesses or physical injuries that could have relevancy to the problems currently facing the patient. By all means, this type of information will also shed great light on social, environmental and cultural conditions which could have greatly influenced the patient during his or her early years, so that one can better understand what is currently happening to the patient. Of course, on many occasions, significant relatives can greatly assist in securing this type of information, and clinicians must try to secure the assistance of the patient's relatives in this regard.

## Sexual History

In the psychiatric field, securing an appropriate sexual history can help tremendously in the analysis and understanding of the patient's present emotional and behavioral problems. For instance, unusual early childhood sexual experiences, the patient and the patient's relatives' perceptions about masturbatory experiences, and sexual preferences and/or dissatisfactions, can all shed light on the patient's problems and conflicts. Certainly, securing this type of information is not an easy task, and therefore, the interviewer must be aware of how much discomfort this type of questioning can bring to both patient and interviewer. However, this discomfort should not constitute an excuse to avoid securing this relevant information. It is through learning and developing adequate skills that clinicians master this difficult but important task.

## Past Medical and Psychiatric History

Obtaining this information can be of great value in assessing what is now happening to a given patient. For instance, one can find out about substance abuse, medications being taken, allergies suffered and the like, all of which can have a direct relationship to the current symptoms and signs being observed in the patient, or to the complaints voiced by him. On other occasions, prior medical illnesses and/or operations such as: venereal diseases, hysterectomies, hyperthyroidism, etc., all can be of great importance in making appropriate differential diagnosis, as well as accurately determining what is currently wrong with the patient in question. Of particular importance here is the obtaining of relevant information about possible past psychiatric problems confronted by the patient. In this regard, this information will not only be of paramount importance in arriving at the correct diagnosis, but will also greatly assist in determining the appropriate treatment, as well as elaboration on the prognostic criteria.

## Family Medical and Psychiatric History

Discovering psychiatric disorders and medical illnesses in the patient's relatives can definitely help in the assessment and evaluation process. In many cases, hereditary medical illnesses such as Huntington's chorea, can be the causative factor in the patient's emotional and/or behavioral problems, and therefore, it is important to eludicate if such a disease has been present among the patient's relatives. In other instances, psychiatric conditions which have been present among the patient's family members such as Manic Depressive Illness can assist the clinician in differentiating among the diagnostic possibilities that could be applied to a given patient since Manic–Depressive Illness is considered to have a potential genetic factor (7, 8). From another standpoint, not only are medical and psychiatric illnesses among the patient's relatives directly related to the patient's condition, but also important events within the family such as suicides, as well as norms and values present in the patient's family mileau such as attitudes towards abortion, religious practices and the like. In other words, the biological, psychological and. socio-cultural relationship between the patient, his family and his total environment can be always perceived by the clinician as having a potential bearing upon the patient's current problems and symptomatology.

## Physical Examination

In every patient displaying behavioral or emotional problems, a thorough physical examination is a must. In many cases, the boundaries between a physical and a mental condition are not only vague, but also difficult to differentiate. It is, therefore, pertinent to rule out all possible physical pathologies which could cause the observed mental symptomatology before one makes a definite psychiatric diagnosis, even in those cases in which it might appear evident that the problems confronted by the patient are only functional in nature. Recent research contributions to the medical literature (9, 10, 11, 12) have greatly influenced the focusing on potential organic factors which can either cause or play a concomitant role in the patient's total psychiatric condition. Of course, this by no means implies that psychological and socio-cultural factors are not important in the determination, presentation and causation of psychiatric disorders.

## Laboratory, Psychological and Ancillary Tests

On many occasions, clinicians have to refer to either laboratory, psychological or other relevant tests such as radiologic procedures, electroencephalography, etc., in order to either rule out a possible organic factor's presence or to confirm a given psychiatric diagnosis. It is therefore important that the clinician be familiar with the use of these tests or have access to a professional who can assist him or her in this regard. Appropriate training and experience will definitely be most helpful in enhancing the clinician's knowledge and skills in this respect. Furthermore, multidisciplinary team approaches in the assessment, diagnosis, treatment determination and follow-up care are also key factors in assuring high quality of care in this regard.

## The Mental Status Examination

The mental status examination represents for the diagnostician the "core" of the armamentarium used in attempting to make a correct diagnosis in a given patient. The mental status examination can be divided into six general sections which I would like to review at this time. They are:

1. *General Appearance and Behavior:* The patient's general appearance and behavior is of great importance in assessing a patient. Much information can be secured from the observation of the patient's general appearance and behavior. For instance, the state of body hygiene, the way in which the patient dresses, his or her mannerisms, facial expressions, body movements, strange postures, reactions to the interview process, display of psychomotor tension and/or anxiety, emotional manifestations of any kind, degree of alertness during the interview and the like, are all major clues which can lead to an accurate psychiatric diagnosis, as well as an understanding of what is happening to the patient.

2. *Characteristics of Speech:* The way in which a patient talks can provide much information in determining what is wrong with him or her. These observed speech pathologies can be defined not only in quantitative terms, but in qualitative terms as well. For instance, a given patient can display a constant and continuous flow in his or her speech pattern in such a way that he or she becomes totally unable to control it. In these types of cases, this pressure of speech and/or flight of ideas can be characteristics of or compatible with a Manic Depressive Illness. On other occasions, the sudden interruption of the speech patterns on a temporary basis can either be a manifestation of "petit mal" epilepsy or of "blocking" phenomenon observed in many schizophrenics, particularly if this interruption in the speech process is accompanied by loosening of associations. In these previously discussed examples, the alteration of the speech process falls into the qualitative aspects of the speech. However, in other cases, the problems lie rather in the qualitative aspects of the speech process. For instance, repetition and return to a given theme within the conversation between patient and clinician, what is known in other words as perseveration, can suggest the presence of organicity in a patient. In other cases, one can observe a certain degree of incoherence, thus suggesting the presence of loosening of association which is observed quite commonly among schizophrenic patients.

Also, neologisms or formation of new words, can also be observed in many cases, which again suggests the presence of a schizophrenic disorder. The crucial point in this regard is that clinicians must pay great attention to all of the qualitative changes or abnormalities in the speech characteristics because they are all important tools in appropriately assessing a patient from a psychiatric point ov view.

3. *Content of Thought:* In every psychiatric examination, the interviewer should encourage a spontaneous development of the patient's mental content. In so doing, the diagnostician will have the opportunity to observe whether misinterpretations of facts and reality is present in an attempt on the patient's part to fulfill his emotional and psychological needs. With some patients, the interviewer should actively ask questions which could help establish the intactness of the patient's content of thought, particularly in patients displaying suspiciousness, defensiveness and lack of cooperation. In these cases, the experience of the interviewer, as well as the rapport already established with these patients, is of paramount importance in being able to successfully insure the patient's trust, confidence and cooperation in this regard. Through this process, the clinician will be able to elucidate if the patient is suffering from a delusion, as well as be able to establish the type of delusions present such as: grandiose delusions, persecutory delusions, somatic delusions, etc. Also, the organization or disorganization of a given delusional system can also be detected. Furthermore, through this process the diagnostician can analyze the presence of obsessive and phobic ideas on the patient's part, as well as dream content, fantasies, ambitions and other important thought content components which can assist in the establishing of an accurate psychiatric diagnosis. Finally, through the examination of the thought content, the clinician can explore for the presence of hallucinatory experiences on the patient's part. In these cases, not only is it important to determine what type of hallucination is present since they can all affect any of the senses such as visual halluciantions, auditory hallucinations, olfactory hallucinations, etc., but also the circumstances in which they are present. These additional details can certainly help in understanding what is wrong with a patient. For instance, hallucinations observed during the time that the patient is trying to get to sleep, generally called hypnagogic hallucinations, take place in healthy

individuals, while auditory hallucinations are commonly seen in schizophrenic disorders, particularly of a paranoid type. Of utmost importance for diagnostic purposes is the elucidation of the presence of any type of hallucinations in a clear sensorium, since in most instances, hallucinations present in a not clear sensorium are the result of toxic or organic conditions.

4. *Mood or Affect:* Manifestations of changes in the mood and/or affect in a person is a good indication of the presence of emotional and psychological disturbances. Of course, one must always keep in mind the circumstances in which these changes take place, as well as the degree of the changes observed before one can label such a change as pathological. In making a psychiatric evaluation, the clinician should try to avoid qualifying the patient's mood as being depressed, elated, euphoric, and the like, but rather, should attempt to describe as clearly as possible how the patient is feeling. This description of the patient's feelings is the best way to elucidate the appropriateness of the mood in relation to the content of thought, as well as the quality and intensity of it. The patient's facial expression and psychomotor tensions are good examples of the type of mood the patient is experiencing. In these cases, the patient's mood is the best representation of the patient's sustained affective state. These mood changes on the patient's part, as well as the manifestations of the affective state on the patient's part are all helpful parameters in determining the patient's psychiatric disorders. For instance, bizarre or inappropriate moods are commonly associated with schizophrenic illnesses while "mood liability," that is, fluctuations in mood in reaction to trivial stimuli, are more often observed in certain types of brain damage. The competent clinician, however, knows that in certain instances, a given mood can be masking a true affective state which is quite different from the type of mood displayed by the patient. For example, with certain patients, manifestations of anger and hostility are nothing else than attempts on the patient's part to deny intense fears of rejection.

5. *Sensorium:* The exploration of the patient's sensorium is the determination of the state of consciousness on the patient's part, as it relates to all of the special senses. In this context, a sensorium can be determined to be clear or clouded in various degrees. These determinations are basic concepts which will assist the clinician in making differential diagnosis and accurate conclusions in respect to a patient's given disturbances. In some patients,

the alterations in the sensorium such as confusion, stupor, etc., might be temporary in nature, thus suggesting, among other things, a toxic state, while in other patients, these manifestations are more or less permanent as seen in cases of dementia. On occasion, a given patient can be so uncooperative and negativistic that the determination of the state of the sensorium has to be delayed as a result of these factors. As part of the sensorium functions, the clinician should determine the grade of orientation in all patients. In this regard, the interviewer should determine if the patient is oriented to person, that is, his own personal identity; to time and to place. Depending on the causation of the patient's psychiatric disorders, the clinician will find different abnormalities in the areas of orientation. For instance, when organic brain damage is the causative factor in determining a given psychiatric condition, the clinician will observe that the patient most often becomes disoriented to either time or place or both. Furthermore, the exploration of the memory functions is also an integral part of the patient's sensorial examination. In this respect, the clinician should examine the patient's capacity to recall remote as well as recent events. Of course, in determining memory functions, particularly of recent nature, and intellectual abilities, the clinician must be aware of the level of education and general interest on the patient's part. For instance, one should not ask a patient to give the name of the best known political figures of the last decade if the patient is a recent migrant to this country, or if he is totally disinterested in political affairs. In other words, the fund of information of the patient must always be taken into consideration when exploring memory functions and intellectual abilities. Insofar as retention and recall abilities, the interviewer must often ask the patient to retain the name of three objects given to him after a lapse of several minutes. In using subtraction of a series of numbers, for instance, seven from a hundred and so on, the clinician can detect the presence of impaired brain functioning. In this respect, it has been reported (13) that 65% of individuals, either healthy persons or mental patients, will offer a correct answer when administered this test. Of course, the patient's education, social class and level of concentration are directly related to his ability to correctly pass this type of test. All of these previously described tests which relate to the functions of the patient's sensorium are extremely useful in characterizing psychiatric conditions along diagnostic classifications, as well as in establishing a realistic treatment plan and a prognostic criteria. Finally, proverb interpretations can also be used within this context as an added test to assist the clinician in arriving at a more conclusive definition of what is wrong with the patient. Again, in using this test, one must take into consideration such factors as level of education, fund of knowledge, intelligence levels, cultural differences, etc. In this respect, generally speaking, schizophrenic patients will offer bizarre interpretations, whereas patients with intellectual impairment will most likely offer concrete interpretations.

6. *Insight and Judgment:* Within the framework of the mental status examination, insight is seen as the patient's capacity to understand and accept that the cause of his or her problems lies in a mental or emotional disturbance. On certain occasions, patients not only will accept this relationship, but can also understand some of the dynamic factors which could play a role in the manifestation of the psychiatric symptomatology. Generally speaking, the greater the insight of a given patient, the greater his potential for a good response to psychodynamically oriented treatment. Insofar as judgment is concerned, while demonstrations of poor judgment do not per se mean presence of mental illness, they do, however, have important diagnostic connotations, as well as influence on the treatment plan to be applied to the patient, and in determining the prognosis. In this context, judgment is seen as the capacity to understand the relationship between a series of related facts and/or ideas, as well as to compare them and arrive at appropriate conclusions about them. Poor judgment in a given case could be the result of both functional factors and organic or toxic factors.


## OVERVIEW OF A DIAGNOSTIC SCHEMA

In this section, I would like to present a general overview of a diagnostic schema in order to provide the readers with a framework from which they can classify most of the clinical cases encountered in their practice. I will not, however, discuss specific disorders within a given diagnostic subgroup since many psychiatric textbooks (14, 15) have already provided this type of information and could readily be used in this regard. In presenting this overview, I will follow the same approach used by the Third

Edition of the Diagnostic and Statistical Manual of Mental Disorders previously aluded to, since this manual represents the most modern and advanced concept in this regard. It is as follows:

## Disorders Usually First Evident in Infancy, Childhood, or Adolescence

This group of disorders is the one observed during infancy, childhood and adolescence. However, there are no well defined age limits in using this type of subclassification of mental disorders. To master the understanding of these disorders, the clinician must know well the stages of normal development. In certain instances, such as with major depressions or schizophrenia, there are no differences in age, and therefore, the diagnosis should be made when the characteristics of the illness in question are found. The mental disorders encountered in this category are:
- Mental Retardation (mild, moderate, severe, profound and unspecified)
- Attention Deficit Disorder (with hyperactivity, without hyperactivity, or residual type)
- Conduct Disorder
    - undersocialized, aggressive
    - undersocialized, nonaggressive
    - socialized, aggressive
    - socialized, nonaggressive
    - atypical
- Anxiety Disorders of Childhood or Adolescence
    - separation anxiety disorder
    - avoidant disorder of childhood or adolescence
    - overanxious disorder
- Other Disorders of Infancy, Childhood or Adolescence
    - reactive attachment disorder of infancy
    - schizoid disorder of childhood or adolescence
    - elective mutism
    - oppositional disorder
    - identity disorder
- Eating Disorders
    - anorexia nervosa
    - bulimia
    - pica

- rumination disorder of infancy
- atypical eating disorder
- atypical eating disorder
— Stereotyped Movement Disorders
  - transient tic disorder
  - chronic motor tic disorder
  - Tourette's disorder
  - atypical tic disorder
  - atypical stereotyped movement disorder
— Other Disorders with Physical Manifestations
  - stuttering
  - functional enuresis
  - functional encopresis
  - sleepwalking disorder
  - sleep terror disorder
— Pervasive Development Disorders
  - infantile autism
  - childhood onset pervasive development disorder
  - atypical pervasive developmental disorder

## Organic Mental Disorders

In this subgroup of disorders, one must include those organic brain syndromes in which the causative factor is either known or presumed. In these disorders, the psychological or behavioral manifestations are the result of temporary or permanent dysfunctions of the brain. The underlying pathophysiological process will determine all of the clinical manifestations observed in these cases. The organic causative factor can either be a primary disease of the brain or a systemic illness that influences the functions of the brain. In this subgroup of disorders, one should include those resulting from substance abuse because of their close relationship to the organic mental disorders. The experienced diagnostician must keep in mind that many of the psychological traits which characterize a person will definitely play a role in the clinical manifestations of the organic mental disorders. Insofar as the Substance Use Disorders in this subgroup, those to be included here are:
- Substance Abuse and Dependence
  - alcohol
  - barbiturate or similar acting sedative or hypnotic

— opioid
— cocaine
— amphetamine or similar acting sympathomimetic
— phencyclidine or similar acting arylcyclohexylamine
— hallucinogen
— cannabis
— tobacco
— other or unspecified substance

In terms of the Organic Mental Disorders, those to be included in this subgroup are:
— Intoxication
— Withdrawal
— Organic Personality Syndrome
— Organic Affective Syndrome
— Organic Hallucinosis
— Organic Amnestic Syndrome
— Delirium
— Dementia
— Atypical or Mixed Organic Brain Syndrome

## Schizophrenic Disorders, Psychotic Disorders Not Elsewhere Classified, and Paranoid Disorders

Most of the mental disorders included in this subgroup will, during the evolution of the illness, show the presence of hallucinations, delusions, severely disorganized behavior and abnormalities in the thinking process and content. In other words, there will be the presence of psychotic features during the active phase of the illness. In these disorders, the causative factors are not related in any way to organic mental disorders or affective disorders. Insofar as schizophrenia is concerned, while a minimal duration of the illness of at least six months is necessary for diagnostic purposes, by no means does this imply that a deteriorating course must be present. In terms of Paranoid Disorders, they are differentiated from Schizophrenia by the absence of prominent hallucinations, incoherence, loosening of associations, or bizarre delusions. In Paranoid Disorders, the main symptomatology is based on persistent persecutory delusions or delusional jealousy not due to any other mental disorders. On occasion, the clinician will observe Psychotic Disorders that can't be classified as either an Organic Mental Disorder, a Schizophrenic, Paranoid or Affective Disorder.

In these instances, the diagnosis to be made is Psychotic Disorders not elsewhere classified. The mental disorders described in this subgroup are:

- Schizophrenic Disorders
    - disorganized
    - catatonic
    - paranoid
    - undifferentiated
    - residual
- Paranoid Disorders
    - paranoia
    - shared paranoid disorder
    - acute paranoid disorder
    - atypical paranoid disorder
- Psychotic Disorders not elsewhere classified
    - schizophreniform disorder
    - brief reactive psychosis
    - schizoaffective disorder
    - atypical psychosis

## Affective Disorders

The primary characteristic of the disorders classified in this subgroup is a disturbance of mood. The abnormalities here could lie in low or high moods. The major categories of this subgroup are the major affective disorders in which one observes a full affective syndrome, other specific affective disorders in which one sees only a partial affective syndrome of at least two years duration, and an atypical affective disorder in which one cannot assign the case to either one of the two previously mentioned categories. In this subgroup the following disorders can be found:

- Bipolar Disorder (mixed, manic, depressed)
- Major Depression (single episode, recurrent)
- Cylothymic Disorder
- Dysthymic Disorder
- Atypical Depression
- Atypical Bipolar Depression

## Anxiety Disorders

In these types of disorders, anxiety is the predominant clinical manifestation. Within this context, anxiety is manifested as:
— Motor Tension: shakiness, jitteriness, trembling, restlessness, etc.
— Autonomic Hyperactivity: sweating, paresthesias, dizziness, cold hands, etc.
— Apprehensive Expectation: fears, worries, anticipation of misfortune to self and others, etc.
— Vigilance and Scanning: hyperattentiveness, impatience, insomnia, lack of concentration, etc.
The disorders classified within this subgroup are:
— Phobic Disorders
  — agoraphobia with panic attacks
  — agoraphobia without panic attacks
  — social phobia
  — simple phobia
— Anxiety States
  — panic disorder
  — generalized anxiety disorder
  — obsessive compulsive disorder
— Post-traumatic Stress Disorder (acute, chronic or delayed)
— Atypical Anxiety Disorder


## Somatoform Disorders

These disorders have as essential features the presence of physical symptoms for which there are no detectable organic illnesses. Different from factitious disorders or malingering, the clinical manifestations in Somatoform Disorders are not under voluntary control. Within this context, the clinician can easily presume that the symptoms are associated with psychological factors. The disorders which fall into this subgroup are:
— Somatization Disorder
— Conversion Disorder
— Psychogenic Pain Disorder
— Hypochondriasis
— Atypical Somatoform Disorder

## Dissociative Disorders

In this subgroup, one will find disorders in which main characteristics are sudden, temporary alteration in the normally integrative functions of consciousness, identity, or motor behavior. Furthermore, one can also observe in these patients an occasional loss of one's own reality which is replaced by a feeling of unreality. In these cases, these findings are in no way due to organic factors or illnesses. The disorders observed in this subgroup are:
- Psychogenic Amnesia
- Psychogenic Fugue
- Multiple Personality
- Depersonalization Disorder
- Atypical Dissociative Disorder

## Psychosexual Disorders

In these disorders, it is understood that psychological rather than organic factors are the determinant or causative factors. Within this context, four major groups compose this category of disorders. The first one is Gender Identity Disorder in which there is an incongruence between anatomic sex and gender identity. The second group is the Paraphilias; in this group the major characteristic factor is the need for unusual or bizarre imagery or acts which must be present in order for a person to obtain sexual excitement. The third group is formed by the Psychosexual Dysfunctions. The essential feature of these disorders is inhibition in the appetitive or psychophysiological changes that characterize the complete sexual response cycle. The fourth one is Other Psychosexual Disorders. A complete review of these four groups shows that the mental disorders encompassed by them are:
- Gender Identity Disorders
  - transsexualism
  - gender identity disorder of childhood
  - atypical gender identity disorder
- Paraphilias
  - fetishism
  - transvestism

- — zoophilia
- — pedophilia
- — exhibitionism
- — voyeurism
- — sexual masochism
- — sexual sadism
- — atypical paraphilia
— Psychosexual Dysfunctions
  - — inhibited sexual desire
  - — inhibited sexual excitement
  - — inhibited female orgasm
  - — inhibited male orgasm
  - — premature ejaculation
  - — functional dyspareunia
  - — functional vaginismus
  - — atypical psychosexual dysfunction
— Other Psychosexual Disorders
  - — ego-dystonic homosexuality
  - — psychosexual disorders not elsewhere classified

## Factitious Disorders

Factitious disorders are those in which the presenting physical or psychological symptoms are under the patient's voluntary control. The clinician assessing these cases must have considerable experience in detecting the fact that the clinical symptomatology is under the patient's voluntary control. However, one must also keep in mind that the presence of a factitious disorder does not rule out the potential co-existence of a physical illness as well. Factitious disorders are to be distinguished from malingering. In malingering, the patient, while having voluntery control of his symptomatology also has a well recognizable main goal in so doing, and full awareness of the circumstances surrounding the case. In Factitious disorders, however, the only goal is for the individual to assume the patient's role. The disorders found within this subgroup are:

- — Factitious Disorders with Psychological Symptoms
- — Chronic Factitious Disorder with Physical Symptoms
- — Atypical Factitious Disorder with Physical Symptoms

## Disorders of Impulse Control Not Elsewhere Classified

These are disorders characterized by:
— Failure to resist an impulse, drive or temptation to perform some act considered harmful to himself or others
— The experiencing of tension before committing the harmful act
— Pleasure and/or sense of relief while committing the harmful act

The categories of disorders found in this subgroup are:
— Pathological Gambling
— Kleptomania
— Pyromania
— Intermittent Explosive Disorder
— Isolated Explosive Disorder
— Atypical Impulse Control Disorder

## Adjustment Disorder

In these disorders, the characteristic feature is a maladaptive reaction to a known psychosocial stressor. The stressor must occur within three months of the presence of the symptomatology. The clinical symptomatology seen is far greater than that which one would expect to see in relation to the given stressor, and leads to social and/or occupational dysfunction on the patient's part. It should be understood that the clinical symptomatology observed can't meet the diagnostic criteria for Anxiety or Affective Disorder. It is also expected that the symptomatology will remit after the disappearance of the causative stressor or stressors. The disorders observed in this subgroup are:
— Adjustment Disorder with Depressed Mood
— Adjustment Disorder with Anxious Mood
— Adjustment Disorder with Mixed Emotional Features
— Adjustment Disorder with Disturbance of Conduct
— Adjustment Disorder with Mixed Disturbance of Emotions and Conduct
— Adjustment Disorder with Work Inhibition
— Adjustment Disorder with Withdrawal
— Adjustment Disorder with Atypical Features

## Psychological Factors Affecting Physical Condition

In many instances, the diagnostician will encounter physholo-gical factors which could either start or exacerbate a given physical condition and/or alter a given symptom's manifestation. In some cases, the patients are totally unaware of the relationship that exists between what is happening in his or her environment and the beginning or changes in a given physical condition and/or symptomatology. Examples of this phenomena can be observed in, among others, asthma, duodenal ulcers, migraine headaches, obesity, and the like. In these cases, the condition can't be the result of a somatoform disorder.

## Personality Disorders

Personality Disorders are those categories resulting from enduring patterns of thinking, feeling and behaving found in a patient in a consistent manner. Furthermore, these given patterns must cause either subjective distress to the patient and/or impair-ment in his or her social and occupational functioning. The dis-orders which fall into this category are not defined as primary ones but rather as secondary in nature. That is, they will be diag-nosed in addition to one of the previously discussed disorders. Within this context they are assigned to the Axis II in the style of diagnosis used in the Third Edition of the Diagnostic and Statisti-cal Manueal of Mental Disorders (DSM-III) previously aluded to. In this category, one should include the following disorders:
— Paranoid Personality
— Schizoid Personality Disorder
— Schizotypal Personality Disorder
— Histrionic Personality Disorder
— Borderline Personality Disorder
— Narcissistic Personality Disorder
— Antisocial Personality Disorder
— Avoidant Personality Disorder
— Dependent Personality Disorder
— Compulsive Personality Disorder
— Passive-Aggressive Personality Disorder
— Atypical Personality Disorder

— Mixed Personality Disorder
— Other Personality Disorder (i.e., Masochistic, Impulsive or Immature Personality Disorder)

## Conditions Not Attributable to a Mental Disorder That Are a Focus of Attention or Treatment

In many cases, the clinician will find that even though a complete assessment has been made on a given patient no mental disorder has been found that could explain the manifestation of his condition. In these cases, one could find that further evaluations and follow–up sometimes lead to the determination of a mental disorder not detected earlier. In these instances, one could make reference to conditions not attributable to a mental disorder. The conditions observed in this subgroup are:
— Malingering
— Borderline Intellectual Functioning
— Adult Antisocial Behavior
— Childhood or Adolescence Antisocial Behavior
— Academic Problem
— Occupational Problem
— Uncomplicated Bereavement
— Noncompliance with Medical Treatment
— Phase of Life Problem or Other Life Circumstance Problem
— Marital Problem
— Parent–Child Problem
— Other Specified Family Circumstances
— Other Interpersonal Problem

## CONCLUSION

In this chapter I have, first of all, tried to demonstrate the importance of a complete psychiatric assessment as the only way of making an accurate diagnosis, and therefore, an appropriate determination of the treatment plan to be applied to a given patient. Secondly, I have reviewed and discussed the psychiatric data base, as well as given special attention to the principles of the mental status examination. Along these lines, I have also tried to provide important and relevant clues and hints which could enhance the experience of the diagnostician in accurately assessing and diagnosing a case. Thirdly, I have presented an overview of a diagnostic schema in accordance with the current use of psychiatric classifications (DSM-III). In this regard, I have tried to assist the clinician and practitioner in appropriately determining what is wrong with the patient and in making  an accurate diagnosis. Hopefully, the material discussed in this chapter will provide the reader with a better understanding of the psychiatric patient, as well as offer an opportunity to further enhance his or her knowledge in the psychiatric field.

# REFERENCES


1. Diagnostic and Statistical Manual of Mental Disorders, Third Edition. Washington, DC: American Psychiatric Association, 1980.

2. Webb LJ, DiClemente CC, Johnstone EE, Sanders JL, Perley RA (Eds.): DSM-III Training Guide. New York: Brunner/Mazel, Publishers, 1981.

3. Fogelson DL, Cohen BM, Pope HG: A study of DSM-III schizophreniform disorders. American Journal of Psychiatry, 139(10):1281-1285, 1982.

4. Craig TJ, Goodman AB, Haugland AG: Impact of DSM-III on Clinical Practice. American Journal of Psychiatry, 139(7):922-925, 1982.

5. Treece C: DSM-III as a research tool. American Journal of Psychiatry, 139(5):577-582, 1982.

6. Skodol AE, Spitzer RL, Williams JBW: Teaching and learning DSM-III. American Journal of Psychiatry, 138(12):1581-1586, 1981.

7. Fieve RR, Mendlewicz J, Fleiss JL: Manic-depressive illness: linkage with Xg blood group. American Journal of Psychiatry, 130:1355-1362, 1973.

8. Allen MG, Cohen S, Pollin W, Greenspan SI: Affective illness in veterans' twins: A diagnostic review. American Journal of Psychiatry, 131(11):1234-1239, 1974.

9. Sachar EG, Frantz AG, Altman N, Sassin M: Growth hormone and prolactin in unipolar and bipolar depressed patients: response to hypoglycemia and L-dopa. American Journal of Psychiatry, 130:1362-1367, 1973.

10. Schildkraut JJ: The catecholamine hypothesis of affective disorders: A review of supporting evidence. American Journal of Psychiatry, 22:507-522, 1965.

11. Harmann E: Longitudinal studies of sleep and dream patterns in manic-depressive patients. Archives of General Psychiatry, 19:311-329, 1968.

12. Coppen A, Eccleston EG, Peet M: Total and free tryptophan concentration in the plasma of depressive patients. Lancet, 2:60-63, 1974.

13. Milstein V, Small JG, Small IF: The substraction of serial sevens test in psychiatry. Archives of General Psychiatry, 26:439-441, 1972.

14 Kolb LC, Brodie HKH: Modern Clinical Psychiatry, Tenth Edition. Philadelphia: W.B. Saunders Company, 1982.

15. Strayhorn, Jr. JM: Foundations of Clinical Psychiatry. Chicago: Year Book Medical Publishers, Inc., 1972.

# Chapter 7

## THE USE OF PSYCHOLOGICAL TESTING: A DIFFERENT WAY TO GET INFORMATION

LOIS C. FRIEDMAN, Ph.D.
JESSE REED, Ph.D.

In this paper, we will address a number of issues relating to psychological tests, their nature and their utility, with special consideration to the needs of the nursing and allied health professions. Among the questions which we will answer are: what is psychological testing; what are the different types of psychological test batteries, and the most commonly used psychological tests; how does psychological testing differ from other ways of assessing patients with known or suspected mental disorders; and how accurate are psychological tests when they are administered to members of different racial, ethnic, and socioeconomic minorities?

## WHAT IS PSYCHOLOGICAL TESTING?

Psychological testing is a type of assessment procedure which is used to obtain systematic samples of verbal, perceptual, and motor behavior under standardized conditions. By "systematic sample" is meant that only a part of a person's behavior is observed, in order to generalize to some characteristic of the individual being assessed; and that in order for this generalization to be valid, the observations must be made in a thorough, regular and methodical, rather than a haphazard or random, manner. The specific behaviors which are observed may already be occurring independent of the assessment procedure, or may be elicited specifically for the purpose of the assessment. In either case, the observations are made (as much as possible) under standardized conditions, in order to minimize the effects of extraneous factors (including the examiner and the environment) upon an individual's test performance.

What is meant by verbal, perceptual, and motor behaviors depends upon the type of psychological evaluation being discussed. Intellectual assessment measures what patients' current levels of intellectual functioning are, and what their premorbid intelligence is likely to have been. Personality assessment is concerned with what kind of psychiatric diagnoses, if any, are suggested; what the nature of patients' conflicts and defenses are; and what the strengths of their character are as well as their weaknesses. Neuropsychological assessment indicates whether there is any evidence for the existence of an organic mental disorder, that is, a dysfunction of the central nervous system. The verbal behavior which is sampled in an intellectual assessment, for example, the extent ot a person's vocabulary, differs from what is relevant verbal behavior for a personality assessment (e.g., responses to the Rorschach ink blot test), which is in turn different from verbal behavior samples in neuropsychological testing (such as the ability to supply the correct name for a number of common, everyday objects). The same holds true for perceptual and, to a lesser extent, motor behavior.

Perceptual acuity (such as in the ability to visually discriminate essential from non–essential detail) is evaluated in intellectual testing; what is perceived when one looks at an ambiguous stimulus (such as an ink blot) is an important source of data for the assessment of personality; and the presence of perceptual distortion (measured, for example, by accuracy of reproduction of a geometric figure) may be an indication of possible brain damage. Similarly, motor speed is involved in the ability to assemble a two–dimensional object from its component parts (intellectual assessment); poor performance on a task involving speed of matching symbols to numbers may, in the absence of brain damage, be a sign of depression (personality assessment); and a greater–than–average difference in grip strength between the right and left hands may help in locating a brain lesion in one or the other cerebral hemispheres (neuropsychological assessment).


## HOW IS PSYCHOLOGICAL TESTING UNIQUE?

Psychologists are not the only mental health professionals who assess patients with mental disorders, nor is psychological testing the only method of assessing such patients. Psychiatrists, neurologists, and nurses, as well as representatives of the various allied health professions, all see patients for the purpose of performing their own particular kind of evaluation. What, then, distinguishes psychological testing from other kinds of patient assessment?

First, psychologists may be the only members of the mental health team who see patients but need not participate directly in their treatment. This is not to say that psychologists never treat patients, or that they do not participate in and contribute to treatment planning; but whereas each of these other health professionals evaluates patients as a first step in treatment, psychologists frequently function primarily as consultants, providing information for others but maintaining a degree of detachment which permits a more considered analysis of  the data, free from the immediate necessity of making treatment decisions.

This same freedom from the immediate concerns of patient care allows psychologists time to investigate certain questions in greater detail than others are able to do. For example, in a neurological examination, physicians must assess not only patient's memories and concentration, but also their reflexes, sensation, gait, balance, and so on; whereas psychologists are able to devote far more time to the measurement of memory in all its aspects, including patients' abilities to remember spatial forms, numbers — both simple and complex —  and familiar and unfamiliar verbal material, etc. As a result, psychologists (especially if they are addressing specific questions about patients) frequently are in a position to gather far more detailed data than others seeing the same patients for different kinds of assessments.

Psychologists also have tools at their disposal which assist them in gathering the data which they use for their evaluations. Just as neurologists, not wishing to rely upon standard electroencephalograms to diagnose (or rule out) seizure disorders, may order sleep–deprived EEGs (because of the effect of sleep deprivation in lowering patients' seizure thresholds), psychologists similarly do not rely upon conversation alone to assess the looseness or tightness of patients' associations, but observe what patients' associations are like, for example, when confronted with the ambiguity of the Rorschach ink blots. And finally, the fact that psychologists gather data in a standardized fashion means that they can make more exact statements by comparing the performance of patients on particular tests to norms (often age-specific norms) which have been developed over long periods of time with large numbers of individuals, both well and ill.

## PSYCHOLOGICAL TESTING AND THE NURSING AND ALLIED HEALTH PROFESSIONS

Because of the great diversity within the allied health professions and the variety of settings in which both nurses and allied health professionals work, a truly thorough consideration of how psychological testing can be meaningful to the nursing and allied health professions would be beyond the scope of this paper. In the most general sense, patient care always is improved when additional information about patients is available to those treating them. However, to bring some order to this, in the concluding section of this paper, we will consider the ways in which nurses and allied helath professionals can utilize psychological test data within our now–familiar typology of psychological tests as intended primarily for either intellectual, personality, or neuro-psychological assessment. All we really are able to do here is supply readers with some hypothetical examples of how psychological test data can be meaningful; they hopefully will have the opportunity to review actual psychological test reports in clinical settings, and to see for themselves how they can enhance their understanding of patients and their problems.

### Intellectual Assessment

Information about patients' intellectual abilities can be useful in a wide variety of ways. Nurses and social workers, for example, may benefit from knowing patients' intellectual levels when judging their reliability as historians for nursing assessments or social histories. Nurses and allied health professional (e.g., dieticians and respiratory therapists) who work with treatment regimens may overestimate patients' intelligence and not appreciate the difficulty which they have in following the regimens prescribed for them; or, alternatively, may underestimate the intelligence of noncompliant patients and attribute their lack of compliance to intellectual inability rather than to motivational or psychodynamic factors. Psychiatric nurses, social workers, art and movement therapists, and others who carry out psychotherapeutic activities with disturbed patients must have an accurate idea of each patient's intelligence in order to judge the patient's capacity for insight, or to tailor their own vocabulary, use of metaphor or analogy in speech, and so on to the intellectual and educational level of each patient, in order not to be misunderstood. In these and many other ways, accurate knowledge of patients' intelligence can greatly improve the quality of patient care offered by nurses and many allied health professionals in both psychiatric and medical/surgical settings; whereas not taking this characteristic into account (or making an "intuitive" but possibly inaccurate estimate of the same characteristic) may lead to misunderstandings and, in some instances to oversights and even to errors in judgment.

## Personality Assessment

The different ways in which knowledge of patients' personality structures can be relevant to nurses and allied health professionals are at least as, and perhaps even more, numerous than is true for information concerning their intellectual functioning. There is scarcely a single aspect of patient care which is not affected by the personalities of the patients being cared for. It is important to realize that under the umbrella of "personality assessment" we are including procedures intended to answer such diverse questions as, for example, whether patients whose logic and reality testing appear seriously impaired suffer from thought disorders (which can be treated with antipsychotic medication) or personality disorders (which cannot); whether patients who complain of depression (or even those who do not, but who show signs of possible depression nevertheless) pose significant suicide risks; what are the patients' formost psychological conflicts and principal defenses against the anxiety engendered by these conflicts; what kinds of symptoms are likely to result if patients' defenses become ineffective; and so on.

The answers to these, and similar, questions are important to those health professionals (nurses and others) who work in psychiatric facilities is most evident. Psychological test reports can provide nurses as well as others (such as occupational and recreational therapists) with information about patients' personalities which may be invaluable in determining the way in which they approach patients and the kinds of activities in which they attempt to involve them, for example, by pointing out difficulties in interpersonal relationships, conflicts over gender identity, or deficiencies in self–esteem. But data on patient's personalities can be equally relevant to medical and surgical settings, to nurses and allied health professionals concerned primarily with providing medical (that is, other than psychiatric) care. Knowing in advance that a particular patient has great difficulty accepting authority may prevent "power struggles" over the administration of medication or the carrying out of certain nursing procedures; and understanding fears which patients who have suffered strokes have of being (or being perceived of as) dependent may make their lack of cooperation with nurses and physical therapists more understandable than it otherwise would be. One could go on and on with similar examples; the point is that nurses and allied health professionals frequently can profit from more information about their patients' personalities, and the best source of such information is likely to be comprehensive psychological evaluations and test reports.

## Neuropsychological Assessment

The third category of psychological tests includes those assessment procedures designed to determine the presence, type, and extent of organic cerebral damage. Brain damage frequently goes unrecognized; and even when it is diagnosed, its effect upon patients' entire psychological states may not fully be understood. Consequently, nurses and allied health professionals may not have the opportunity to help such patients to the extent that they could if the results of neuropsychological assessments were available.

Brain damage may affect patients in a variety of ways. Focal (i.e., specific and localized) lesions, for example, may seriously compromise one or more mental ability, while leaving others largely or completely unimpaired. Nurses who work with brain-damaged patients in hospitals, rehabilitation centers and nursing homes; occupational and corrective therapists who plan and administer activities directed toward the maintenance or restoration of functions; speech pathologists whose objective is the restoration of communication skills; social workers and discharge planning nurses who are concerned with how patients adjust to their environments following discharge — all these will benefit from exact knowledge of what brain-injured patients are (and are not) capable of doing. Diffuse (i.e., generalized) brain damage is frequently less than obvious; also, some patients with impaired memory or reasoning ability appear normal superficially, but formal neuropsychological examination may indicate the presence of deficits which have significant, although subtle, effects upon their ability to function cognitively.

Finally, brain damage may have yet another kind of effect — upon emotions — which nurses and allied health professionals must understand if they are to work effectively with brain-injured patients. Patients' emotional states may be affected in direct ways, as in Organic Affective Syndrome, in which symptoms of depression, hypomania, or emotional lability result from organic impairment itself; or the emotional effects may be indirect, as in those patients whose awareness of their own deficits (particularly in areas of functioning which are utilized regularly and frequently, such as memory) become the source of depression, irritability and anger. This latter kind of effect is, unfortunately, too often overlooked; it is presumed that organic deficits are accompanied by a lack of awareness (the "they don't know the difference" attitude); or the organic deficits are so subtle that their significance is not realized or appreciated by anyone except the patients themselves, whose efforts to express their increasing feelings of incapacity may be met with indifference or denial. It is important to recognize that patients frequently are aware of even slight changes in their mental capabilities; that the significance of such changes depends upon their premorbid personalities and levels of functioning (for example, even a slight decline in numerical recall may be far more threatening to a former accountant than a larger decline in the same ability might be to a painter or poet); and that only by being aware of the existence, nature and extent of such deficits can health professionals working with brain-injured patients appreciate the emotional effects of their impairments, and assist them in make more adequate adjustments.

# PSYCHOLOGICAL TESTS MOST FREQUENTLY USED

The purpose of this section is to acquaint the reader with some of the more frequently utilized tests in each of the three principal areas of psychological evaluation (see Table I for a list of the major intellectual, personality, and neuropsychological tests). This is not intended to be a comprehensive review of available psychological tests. Instead, a number of representative tests, selected on the basis of their frequency of use, will be described, these being the tests most likely to be referred to in psychological test reports.

## Intellectual Assessment

The purpose of intellectual testing is to assess intelligence. The results (usually expressed as IQ scores) compares current levels of functioning to what is average for persons of similar age (normative expectations).

---

**TABLE I**
**MAJOR PSYCHOLOGICAL TESTS**

| | |
|---|---|
| INTELLECTUAL | Stanford–Binet |
| | Wechsler Preschool and Primary Scale of Intelligence (WPPSI) |
| | Wechsler Intelligence Scale for Children (WISC) |
| | Wechsler Adult Intelligence Scale (WAIS) |
| PERSONALITY | Minnesota Multiphasic Personality Inventory (MMPI) |
| | Cattell Sixteen Personality Factor Questionnaire (16PF) |
| | Rorschach Inkblot Test |
| | Thematic Apperception Test (TAT) |
| NEUROPSYCHOLOGICAL | Wechsler Memory Scale (WMS) |
| | Luria–Nebraska Neuropsychological Battery |
| | Halstead–Reitan Neuropsychological Battery |

---

Intelligence is not a single or unitary ability; consequently, intelligence tests measure a number of different skills. Most tests divide skills into verbal and nonverbal areas (sometimes referred to as Verbal and Performance tests), which are thought to correspond roughly to the left and right hemispheres of the brain, respectively. In addition to obtaining overall IQ scores and to comparing different specific abilities, psychologists often learn a great deal about patients' personalities by looking at such qualitative aspects of their test performance as the manner in which they approach and execute tasks, the way in which they react to frustration or failure, and so on.

The most widely used tests of intelligence are the *Stanford–Binet* test and the three *Wechsler* tests (one test for pre-school children, one for school–age children, and one for late adolescents and adults). The Stanford–Binet (originally the Binet–Simon) was first published in 1908 as a test of children's intelligence, and was revised in 1911 for use with adults as well. Although still in use, the Stanford–Binet is generally less popular than the Wechsler tests becuase psychologists must continue testing until their patients fail all the items at a particular age leve (to establish a test "ceiling"), a procedure which sometimes makes administration of the test extremely lengthy.

There are three Wechsler tests: the Wechsler Preschool and Primary Scale of Intelligence (WPPSI); the Wechsler Intelligence Scale for Children (WISC); and the Wechsler Adult Intelligence Scale (WAIS). The last two recently have been published in revised forms as the WISC-R and WAIS-R, respectively. Although the tasks and items on the three tests obviously are different, so as to be suitable for the three different age groups for which they are intended, the basic structure of each of the three tests is the same. Each test is divided into Verbal and Performance subtests, the former measuring such areas as general knowledge about the world; ability to reason abstractly; vocabulary; judgment in everyday situations; and basic arithmetic skills. The Performance subtests include speed of matching numerals and abstract symbols (on the WPPSI, the task involves matching colors to animals, in order to be appropriate for preschoolers); abstract spatial reasoning; visual perceptiveness; and concrete spatial abilities. In addition to giving total ("Full Scale") IQ scores and separate Verbal and Performance IQ's, norms are available so that individuals' scores on each subtest can be compared to what is "average" for their age.

Although the Stanford-Binet test is still used in educational settings (particularly with intellecutally impaired children), the Wechsler tests (most commonly the WAIS-R and WISC-R) are the most frequently utilized in clinical settings.

Other tests of intelligence are available for general or specialized uses. The *Shipley-Institute of Living Scale* is a self-administered test of vocabulary and abstract reasoning. The *Ammons Quick Test* and the *Peabody Picture Vocabulary Test* take only a few mintues to administer, although they give no information on different dimensions of intelligence. The *Leiter* is particularly well suited to the examinaiton of deaf persons or persons with whom language barriers exists, since it is entirely non-verbal, requiring no instructions (except by example) and no verbal questions or replies.

## Personality Assessment

Personality assessment techniques include a variety of tests intended to identify, describe and classify peoples' emotional, motivational, interpersonal and attitudinal characteristics. These techniques may be grouped into two general categories: objective self-report instruments and projective tests. Although some personality tests are used for group screening purposes, most are used in clinical and counseling settings.

*Objective self-report instruments* consist of a list of standardized items, which are answered by choosing among two or more alternatives. The best known and most widely used of these is the *Minnesota Multiphasic Personality Inventory* (MMPI). It consists of 566 statements which are answered either "True" or "False." The statements cover a wide range of content areas, including health, psychosomatic symptoms, social and political attitudes, past experiences, and various indications and manifestations of neurotic and psychotic disturbances.

Appropriate for late adolescents and adults, the MMPI originally was intended to assist in establishing psychiatric diagnoses. This was done by developing different scales (combinations of items answered in particular ways) which were found to be empirically related to specific psychiatric disorders. Research on the uses of the MMPI has been extremely extensive; so that rather than simply suggesting psychiatric diagnoses, MMPI profiles (the configuration of scores on the various scales) help psychologists form pictures of patients' personalities, including such things as their underlying dynamics, levels of adjustment, contact with reality, characteristic defenses, and likely behaviors in different kinds of situations (1). The MMPI is an extremely useful instrument in both general medical and psychiatric settings, and is frequently utilized as a screening device for certain kinds of psychopathology, to provide initial assessments of new patients, as an aid in the development of treatment plans, and to evaluate progress during and following psychiatric treatment.

The ten clinical scales of the MMPI are: hypochondriasis; depression; hysteria; psychopathy; masculinity–femininity; paranoia; psychasthenia (anxiety); schizophrenia; hypomania; and social introversion. Three scales are used for assessing the validity, or meaningfulness, of each profile. The normal value for each of the scales is known, and interpretations of MMPI profiles are based upon the extent to which scores on any of the scales exceeds the normal range, as well as upon the specific combination of above-normal scales.

Another well known objective test of personality is the *Cattell Sixteen Personality Factor Questionnaire* (16 PF). Unlike the MMPI, the 16 PF was developed using a normal population, and is not intended to identify psychopathology or establish psychiatric diagnoses. Rather, it gives a picture of personality in terms of basic dimensions, or traits, such as: reserved–outgoing; humble–assertive; shy-venturesome; and others. Because it does not deal with categories of psychopathology, the 16 PF (like similar tests, such as the *Eysenck Personality Inventory*) is less frequently employed in clinical settings than is the MMPI.

*Projective tests* are distinguished from objective self–report instruments by the unstructured nature of the tasks. In contrast to the specific questions asked on objective tests, projective tests consist of ambiguous stimuli; patients are given only the briefest possible instructions; and the free use of their imaginations is encouraged. The fundamental assumption of all projective techniques is that the ways in which people perceive and interpret the ambiguous stimuli which make up these tests reveal various aspects of the structure and functioning of their personalities, including the nature of their fantasy lives, their anxieties and defenses, the adequacy of their reality testing, and how they operate in unstructured or stressful situations.

Two of the most widely used projective tests are the *Rorschach Test* and the *Thematic Apperception Test* (TAT). The Rorschach, originated by a Swiss psychiatrist in 1921, consists of ten cards, each showing a bilaterally symmetrical inkblot. Seven of the designs (all of which are printed on white backgrounds) are entirely or primarily in different shades of gray, while three are in pastel colors. Patients are shown the cards one at a time and are asked what each of the designs could be; after they have given as many responses to each of the cards as they want to, they are asked to elaborate upon each of their responses and to explain what made it look like what it did.

Although there are several systems for scoring Rorschach records (2, 3), the use of a formal system is not required for interpretation. Such aspects of the record as the total number of responses; responsiveness to color in the inkblots; the way in which different parts of an inkblot are (or are not) integrated into a meaningfully organized response; the responsiveness to shapes (how easily, if at all, others are able to perceive what patients see); and the content of the responses (for example, whether they are morbid and bizarre, or fearful, or lively and animated, or highly sexual) all enter into the interpretations which psychologists make of Rorschach records.

Probably the next most frequently utilized projective test is the *Thematic Apperception Test,* or TAT. Similar tests also exist for certain restricted age groups, such as the Children's Apperception Test for preschool and early school age children; the Michigan Pictures Test for latency age children; the Symonds Picture Story Test for adolescents; and the Senior Apperception Test for the elderly; but the principle of each of these tests is the same, and only the TAT will be discussed here.

The TAT is a more structured test than the Rorschach. It consists of a set of drawings of people, alone or in pairs or groups. Patients make up a story to go with each picture they are shown; and they are then asked to elaborate on certain aspects of their stories (for example, what is happening in the drawing; what the thoughts and/or feelings of the people in the picture appear to be; and how the story is going to end). No specified number of combination of pictures is shown to patients; most psychologists select from eight to twelve pictures, the specific ones depending upon patients' personal characteristics (such as age, sex, and marital status) and the dynamic and/or diagnostic questions which psychologists wish to answer. The pictures deal with a variety of intrapersonal and interpersonal themes, among them parent-child, sibling, heterosexual and homosexual relationships; frustration, achievement, loneliness and depression; and aggression, intimacy, nurturance and dependence. The nature and content of patients' fantasies about each picture are used as a basis for making inferences about different aspects of their personalities; their relationships with significant people in their lives, both past and present; and the way in which they are likely to behave in a variety of situations.

## Neuropsychological Assessment

Although there are a large number of individual tests designed for the purpose of differentiating between neurologically impaired and unimpaired persons, the complexity of the human brain is such that a battery of tests is far more effective than any single test in identifying brain damage and specifying the location and extent of injury of the brain. The two most widely used test batteries of this type are the *Luria-Nebraska* and the *Halstead-Reitan* neuropsychological batteries. For reasons of economy of space, only the second of these will be described in this paper.

The Halstead-Reitan battery is a group of tests which, used in combination, provides a systematic way of inferring the presence, severity, and localization of brain damage. Diagnosis of the presence and severity of brain damage is made by comparing patients' scores on the component tests with established norms, as well as with their estimated premorbid functioning, inferred from such information as their educational and occupational achievements. Diagnosis of the localization of brain damage is based upon differences in performance on different parts of the test battery, since the tests making up the battery were chosen to measure the functioning of each of the areas of the cerebral cortex.

The Wechsler Adult Intelligence Scale (WAIS, or WAIS-R) is a fundamental part of the Halstead-Reitan battery. This test, which has already been described in detail earlier in this paper, provides a baseline measure of current intellectual functioning; given information on premorbid intellectual ability (since some subtests are more subject than others to the effects of organic impairment); provides a rough comparison of the functioning of the right and left hemispheres of the brain; and assesses specific areas of cognitive functioning known to be associated with certain areas of the brain, such as arithmetic reasoning, visual–spatial skill, and others.

Another component test of the Halstead–Reitan battery is the Wechsler Memory Scale (WMS), a test which often is used independently of the entire battery (sometimes in combination with the WAIS or WAIS–R) as well. The WMS assesses orientation to time and place; awareness of current events; performance of rote mental tasks (such as reciting the alphabet, counting backwards, and counting by three's); and the ability to both recall and retain numbers, words, simple paragraphs and geometric forms. The result of this test is expressed in a score (the Memory Quotient), which is similar  to an IQ score in that it is adjusted for patients' ages and varies around an average score of 100.

In addition to the WAIS (or WAIS–R) and the WMS, the Halstead–Reitan battery includes a test of concept formation; tests measuring recognition of differences in rhythmic patterns and nonsense syllables; a task in which patients connect a series of circles in alternating sequences of letters and numbers (i.e., A→1→ B→2, etc.); a comparison of fine motor coordination in the dominant and non–dominant hands; a measure  of the ability to place variously shaped wooden blocks in holes of the same shapes while blindfolded, both with the dominant and non–dominant hands; a test of sensory functioning (especially the sense of touch); and a survey of signs of receptive and expressive aphasia (inability to comprehend spoken language and to express oneself verbally), dyslexia (inability to understand the written word), dysgraphia (inability to write), dyscalculia (inability to do arithmetic tasks), dysarthria (inability to repeat words out loud) and dyspraxia (inability to perform certain motor tasks and to follow instructions). A careful comparison of the patients' levels of functioning on each of the various tests making up the Halstead Reitan battery, including those on which the performance of the dominant and non–dominant hands are compared, can indicate not only the presence of brain damage, but also whether the damage is diffuse or localized; whether it is lateralized, and if so, in which hemisphere; and (if it is not diffuse) in what region of the cerebral cortex it is likely to exist.

## PSYCHOLOGICAL TESTING AND MINORITY PATIENTS

The validity of using psychological test procedures with persons whose racial, ethnic, or socioeconomic backgrounds are different from those of the persons used in the standardization of these tests has been in question since prior to World War I (4). In fact, the United States Army even developed a non-verbal test of intelligence at that time, in order to evaluate the capabilities of recruits from rural areas who had had little or no formal education (5). Since then, many studies have shown differences in intelligence test scores between children from higher and lower socioeconomic backgrounds and between white and black children; and social class differences in responses to projective tests, such as the Rorschach, have also been found (6). Cultural and sub-cultural differences easily can become disadvantages when people must compete within cultural contexts other than those in which they were raised; and psychological tests, therefore, inevitably are likely to favor persons from the dominant culture, within which the tests were developed and standardized.

There are several ways in which psychological tests may discriminate against persons from racial, ethnic, and socioeconomic minorities. The content of the items on many standardized tests (both intelligence and objective personality tests) frequently are biased to reflect middle-class white culture. Language styles (including the meaning attributed to certain words or phrases) also differ; and minority patients may be at a disadvantage not only in understanding what is required of them, but also in the manner in which they express their responses, which may be misunderstood or misinterpreted by psychologists who neither share nor understand minority patients' cultural and linguistic backgrounds. Furthermore, some of the tasks involved in certain psychological assessment procedures may be less familair to minority patients; some of the test materials may be less meaningful to them; and they may be less comfortable (and therefore may perform differently) when examined by psychologists whose ethnic backgrounds are different from their own. Although these factors do not invalidate the use of psychological tests with minority patients, they do suggest that the results of such tests should be interpreted with an extra measure of caution in order to insure that cultural differences are not mistakenly seen as indicators of intellectual limitation or personality pathology.

## SUMMARY

In this paper, the nature and purpose of psychological testing have been defined; the way in which psychological evaluation differs from psychiatric assessment has been explained; and the relevance of the results of these tests to nurses and allied health professionals has been demonstrated. Several of the most frequently utilized tests from each of the three basic categories of psychological assessment procedures — intellectual, personality, and neuropsychological assessment — have been described as well. Finally, a word of caution was added regarding the validity of using psychological tests with members of minority groups, when these tests have been standardized primarily on non-minority persons, and may reflect the content and values of the dominant culture in a variety of ways. Understanding what psychological testing is, and how and why psychological tests are used, will enable nurses and allied health professionals to derive the maximum amount of information into their own activities in order to improve the quality of the care which they provide their patients.

## REFERENCES

1. Golden CJ: Clinical Interpretation of Objective Psychological Tests. New York: Grune & Stratton, 1979.

2. Exner JE: The Rorschach: A Comprehensive System. New York: John Wiley and Sons, 1974.

3. Allen RM: Student's Rorschach Manual. New York: International Universities Press, 1973.

4. Abel TM: Psychological Testing in Cultural Contexts. New Haven, CT: College and University Press, 1973.

5. Haney W: Validity, vaudeville, values: A short history of social concerns over standardized testing. American Psychologist, 36:1021-1034, 1981.

6. Friedman LC, Patterson, GK, Gomez RR: A socioeconomic minority: The poor and mental health care. The American Journal of Social Psychiatry, Vol. 3(2):19-25, 1983.

# Chapter 8

## MENTAL HEALTH EMERGENCIES: RECOGNIZING IMMEDIATE DANGERS

RANJIT C. CHACKO, M.D.
LAWRENCE ROOT, M.D.

A mental health emergency is one in which an abrupt disruption in homeostasis occurs because of a biological, psychological, or social event, which has modified the patients' mood, thinking or behavior to such an extent that the patient and/or the ones seeking help on his/her behalf believe that there is an urgent need for intervention.

## INTRODUCTION

In the past 15 years, emergency psychiatry services in the United States have experienced a phenomenal growth in availability and utilization (1). This growth has produced both positive and negative effects in terms of mental health service delivery. Psychiatric emergency services now serve as critical entry points into a network of community mental health services. They are often the sole source of treatment for many deinstitutionalized chronically mentally ill patients due to the lack of alternative treatment settings in the community. The number of younger patients seeking emergency psychiatry services have also shown dramatic increases in the past two decades (1). Alcohol and drug related problems such as intoxication, withdrawal and the medical and psychological complications of prolonged substance abuse are frequently encountered in emergency rooms. In addition, due to the inadequacy of third party reimbursement for ambulatory mental health services, psychiatric emergency rooms serve as the only resource for the poor and indigent mentally ill.

Mental health emergencies are encountered in a variety of clinical settings. Traditional settings include professional's offices, general hospital emergency rooms, community mental health centers, state hospitals, nursing homes and correctional facilities. The adequate handling of an acutely disturbed psychiatric patient requires certain modifications to the architecture of conventional clinical settings (2). For example, the acute psychotic patient needs a larger body–buffer zone of safety to be comfortable and non-threatened by the presence of other patients. Also, larger doorways for ready exit from interview rooms and fixed furniture often provides the simple additional security measures that are not available in many treatment facilities.

The staff of a psychiatric emergency service is generally multidisciplinary in nature. A variety of professionals with highly specialized skills work together in teams to provide the comprehensive assessment and treatment that is required in such crisis situations. The staff/patient ratio is also generally much higher than on the average inpatient treatment service. Psychiatrists, emergency room physicians, psychiatric nurses, psychologists, social workers, allied health professionals and other support staff must work together as cohesive teams to meet the complex needs of the psychiatric patient in crisis. Instead of a calm, empathic, listening and inquiring atmosphere, emergency services often are designed to the rapid containment and resolution of only life threatening situations — rapid assessment and rapid disposition (3, 4). As a result, the relationship between patient and therapist usually suffer irreversible damage. A number of studies have clearly shown that extended emergency evaluations actually decrease hospitalization rates and increase the acceptance of treatment referrals by patients (5, 6). The goal of the psychiatric staff is twofold: 1) evaluate and treat the identified patient, 2) reassure and educate the significant others as to their role in the treatment and rehabilitation of the patient. The family members' anxiety often stems from guilt (conscious or unconscious) over their contribution to the development of the crisis. The family guilt/anxiety may be manifested by a defensive attitude, a sense of urgency that something has to be done immediately, open hostility towards the staff or sometimes even apathy. In these types of situations, at times it is difficult for the staff to remain calm, non-judgmental, understanding and project the appearance that they can and will help the patient with the problem. As a general rule, there are few psychiatric emergencies that demand immediate action before one has time to gather data, and develop an understanding of the problem before treatment is initiated. It is essential that each staff member be aware of their own limitations in dealing with a crisis, and request assistance from others whenever they are exceeded.

## SUICIDAL BEHAVIOR

Suicidal behavior is characterized by the attempt to take one's own life or by activities that put a person in a precarious situation so that the risk of death or injury to themselves is increased. Suicidal behavior most commonly occurs in patients who are depressed, but can also be seen in patients with other psychotic disorders, organic brain syndromes, and character disorders.

### General Principles in the Evaluation of Suicidal Patients

As a rule, suicidal behavior increases with age. Men are more successful in their attempts than women (3:1) but women attempt suicide more frequently (3:1) (7). Single persons are twice as likely to successfully commit suicide, and divorced or widowed persons are four to five times more likely to kill themselves (7). Caucasian protestants have a higher rate of suicide and homosexuals have higher rates than heterosexuals (7).

Two sets of overlapping suicidal patient populations are encountered: 1) those who attempt suicide, few of whom go on to commit it, and 2) those who commit suicide many of whom previously have attempted it. The ratio between suicide attempts and

---

**TABLE I**
**HIGH RISK FACTORS FOR SUICIDE**

Males
Age Ranges: 15–21 years     55–70 years
Caucasians
Single
Widowed
Divorced
Past History of Suicide Behavior
Family History of Suicide
History of Alcohol or Substance Abuse
History of Major Affective Disorders

---

actual suicides is 8 to 1 (7). The lethality of the suicidal attempt is an important consideration. The more violent the route of suicide the higher the risk, i.e., gunshot wounds, jumping from high places, hanging, vs. overdoses or slashing wrists (8). Seventy percent of patients who commit suicide have seen a physician within four months of their suicide, and have expressed suicidal ideations (7).

## Risk Factors in the Depressed Patient

This category constitutes the largest number of patients who successfully commit suicide. There is usually a family history of suicide, depression or alcoholism. Patients at highest risk are those who exhibit a retarded type of major depression, with prominent insomnia, anorexia, weight loss, hopelessness and strong guilt feelings. One should be particularly suspicious of patients with a history of depression who suddenly begin giving away cherished possessions, change their life insurance policies or write new wills (8). Most suicides occur within three months after the onset of recovery in depression (7).

Depressive illness is often triggered by a real loss or a threatened loss. The losses may be social (divorce, separation, death of a relative, lost custody of children), financial (unemployment, bankruptcy) or physical (loss of physical health, debilitating illness, plastic surgery). This type of stress is particularly a problem if it affects the person's independence, and takes away a person's reason to live. The patient then contemplates suicide as the only way out of a hopeless dilemma.

## Risk Factors in the Psychotic Patient

These individuals in many ways are at the highest risk because their behavior is erratic and unpredictable. The psychotic patient who is delusional and experiences command hallucinations regarding suicide is in urgent need of hospitalization and close observation. For example, a paranoid schizophrenic may hear voices directing the patient to walk across a busy freeway. Patients who are delusional and guilt ridden are prone to kill themselves, especially if they experience condemnatory auditory hallucinations. Manic bipolar patients and excited catatonic patients also require supervision and treatment because their behavior often incites others to harm them or act out in an impulsive and reckless manner which may result in severe injury and/or death.

## Risk Factors in the Organic Patient

The organic patient invariably has deficiencies in judgment. Organicity also seems to lower control over one's own impulses and produces aggressive and violent outbursts of behavior. The most frequent cause of organicity leading to suicidal behavior is alcohol and drug intoxication. It is estimated that in at least 50% of the suicides, alcohol has been a major contributing factor (7). Certain hallucinogens like PCP have also been reported to produce bizarre suicide attempts. Patients with chronic brain damage due to senile dementia, post head injury or stroke patients can have their judgment so impaired that they accidently kill themselves by wandering out into traffic, or inadvertently poison themselves by taking prescribed medication improperly.

## Risk Factors in Personality Disorder Patients

Patients with certain types of personality disorders engage repeatedly in self–destructive behavior usually in response to stress. Patients with borderline personality disorders for example, frequently threaten to kill themselves in order to manipulate significant others. Even though their attempts are not as lethal, the frequent attempts produce a higher risk for "unintentional suicide." Antisocial, narcissistic, compulsive, and histrionic patients are also at higher risk for suicidal behavior.

## Management of the Suicidal Patient

The management of suicidal behavior is dependent upon the associated psychiatric illness and psychosocial precipitants. However, as a general rule, severely suicidal paitents are never left unattended before, during, or after an evaluation. Patients who have suicidal ideations and a psychosis, might be hospitalized and treated with antipsychotic and antidepressant medications until their psychotic thinking has been ameliorated. In some instances, electro–convulsive therapy is necessary for rapid resolution of a major depression with severe suicidal ideation. Patients who are intoxicated and suicidal must be hospitalized until their intoxication subsides, and they regain better control over their impulses and judgment. Patients who have deteriorating brain disease require custodial care in a nursing or foster home in order to protect them from themselves. Suicidally depressed patients generally experience brief periods of high suicidal intentionality that usually last only for a few hours or days. Patients are therefore hospitalized and observed for a period of at least 24 hours and preferably three days, subsequent to a suicide attempt (9). Antidepressant medication can be initiated while the patient is in the hospital, and plans should be made with the family for follow-up treatment and psychotherapy. It is unwise to return a patient to the same environment that contributed to his suicidal state without a thorough investigation and assessment of these stressors.

## ASSAULTIVE BEHAVIOR

As a general rule, assaultive behavior is usually handled by correctional facilities. Yet, many patients seek psychiatric assistance because they feel they are going to loose control of their own impulses or explode violently. There are other patients who become assaultive as a direct result of psychotic or organic mental disorders that interfere with their ability to test reality and control their own aggressive impulses. In this latter group of patients, the risk of sudden unprovoked violence is high.

### General Principles in the Evaluation of an Assaultive Patient

The most important aspect of the interview is that the interviewer have a calm and firm sense that he/she can and will help the assaultive patient control their own impulses. An interviewer who feels out of control will only exacerbate anxiety and agitation in the patient. In these instances, immediate assistance must be sought from colleagues or supervisors (10).

Assaultive behavior is often manifested by increased volume and intensity of speech, threatening comments, gestures, and psychomotor agitation. The patient may get up and begin walking around or pacing up and down the room and exhibit a startle response. These last two signs often signal imminent loss of control (10).

It is important that the patient is treated in a calm and respectful manner (e.g., addressing the patient in a formal manner — Mr. or Mrs. A.) and spoken to in a nonjudgmental fashion. If possible, one should attempt to assume the same level of eye contact (for example, stand until the patient sits down). The staff should not conduct an interview with an armed patient under any circumstances. All patients suspected of carrying weapons should be searched prior to the interview. Weapons should not be taken from the patient directly but instead the patient is asked to place the weapon on the floor or table in front of them (10). If the interviewer still feels uncomfortable, a security guard should be requested. The interviewer should never position himself away from an available exit. The interview must be conducted in a quiet room with adequate space so as to not feel cramped (1). Do not touch or examine the patient physically without permission, and respect the patient's right to refuse physical examination unless it is absolutely necessary. Sudden or quick moves are avoided. Do not provoke the patient, and allow enough time for the patient to respond to questions. If the interviewer is unable to develop rapport with the patient, a family member or friend should be asked to assist in the interview (10).

## Management of the Assaultive Patient

The primary goal in the management of the assaultive patient is to re-establish within the patient some sense of impulse control. Assaultive patients require structure and rigid limits set on their aggressive behavior (11).

The treatment and management of such a patient begins with the establishment of rapport through an empathic and nonjudgmental approach by the therapist. Reassurance, understanding and a calm acceptance of the patient's anger and rage is usually enough to reduce the tension to the point where practical measures can be taken to deal with acute impulses.

Physical restraints are required when the physician is unable to establish this rapport with an agitated patient, and the patient refuses to cooperate with verbal commands to control his agitation or take medications (10). In order to adequately and safely restrain a patient, it takes at least five staff members — one for each limb, and one to apply the restraints and/or administer medications (12). Restraints should be applied in a firm fashion without argument or bargaining with the patient. The patient is informed that restraints are necessary for his own protection and that it is only a temporary measure. Once the patient is in restraints, rapid tranquilization with antipsychotics is often utilized to calm the patient down so that his restraints can be removed as soon as possible (13). Seclusion rooms should also be used in a similar manner with frequent re-evaluation of the patient. Medication is used to reduce psychotic thinking or to treat withdrawal states (i.e., opiate withdrawal or D.T.'s). When medication is administered, the patient should always be given the choice to take it by injection, or by mouth preferably in liquid concentration form. There should be some verbal reassurances that the medication will help to calm the patient (13).

## THE ORGANICALLY IMPAIRED PATIENT

The organic patient may present to an emergency service with either a delirium (acute brain syndrome) or with a dementia (chronic brain syndrome). Patients with organic brain syndromes, exhibit deficits in higher mental functioning such as memory, orientation, abstraction, concentration and judgment. There may also be disturbances in sensorium, perception, mood and thinking.

Delirium usually develops fairly quickly, frequently within hours or days. It is generally caused by some external agent (drugs, alcohol, head trauma, withdrawal syndromes) or due to some internal medical derangement (metabolic, infectious or vascular problems). If these causes can be diagnosed and reversed before permanent damage to the brain develops, then dementia is prevented from developing.

Dementia usually presents with an insidious onset and a progressive course. Dementia may be due to an irreversible condition such as Alzheimer's nutritional anemia. Therefore, the careful assessment of the demented patient is necessary, and a thorough physical examination and laboratory investigation is required.

## Guidelines to the Evaluation of an Organic Patient

A standard and routine procedure for the comprehensive assessment of patients suffering from organic brain syndromes should be available at all emergency centers. The process generally involves a multidisciplinary team of professionals and follows a rigid structured format for investigation. Clues leading to the diagnosis of an organic brain syndrome will emerge from a detailed psychiatric history and mental status examination. The goals of the assessment process are twofold: 1) the differentiation of delirium from dementia; 2) the identification of a specific etiologic agent that has produced the organic symptomatology, particularly if treatment is available to arrest or reverse the disease process itself.

The following steps are useful guidelines in the management of patients who present with "organic mental disorders." Obviously, all steps will not necessarily be used in the assessment of every patient due to time and cost factors: 1) A detailed psychiatric history which specifically includes information regarding developmental history, precipitating stressors, and family history. 2) A detailed medical history that includes information regarding alcohol or other substance abuse, head trauma, exposure to toxic substances and a list of all current medications. 3) Complete physical examination that includes a neurological assessment. 4) Neuropsychological testing to assess the degree of organicity and identify specific focal pathology. 5) Laboratory studies — CBC, SMAC, thyroid function tests, $B_{12}$ and folate levels, VDRL, drug and toxic substance screening. 6) Chest and skull x–rays. 7) EEG. 8) EKG. 9) CSF studies. 10) CAT scan.

## Management of an Organic Patient

The first step in the management of an organic patient is to identify an etiological agent by using a comprehensive assessment procedure as outlined above. Next, a specific treatment that either arrests or reverses the disease process is instituted as quickly as possible before further brain damage occurs. In general, no sedating neuroleptic drugs should be administered to patients under investigation, especially in cases of delirium where the level of consciousness often becomes the only indicator of a deteriorating condition. Patients are treated intensively for their medical conditions, monitored closely and life support systems are used to tide them over the crisis period if necessary. In some cases, small dosages of antipsychotic agents (low dose, high potency drugs like haloperidol, fluphenazine) or benzodiazepines (diazepam) are used in the management of severe psychomotor agitation especially if this behavior interferes with the medical management óf the patient thus endangering life.

## THE PSYCHOTIC PATIENT

Psychotic behavior is symptomatic of several general types of mental illnesses, and is characterised by a loss of reality testing, disorganization of personality, disturbances in mood, thinking, perception, and sometimes, memory judgment, orientation, and intellect. Psychotic behavior is often violent, bizarre and irrational and obviously "crazy."

Psychotic disorders can be categorized into two general subgroups — the functional and the organic psychoses. Functional psychoses presents with marked distrubances in mood, affect, thinking and perception with usually no deficits in orientation, memory or intellect. The category of functional psychoses include disorders such as schizophrenia, manic depressive illness and paranoid disorders. Organic psychoses can resemble functional psychoses in all respects, except that the most outstanding features are deficits in memory, intellect and orientation. Organic psychoses by definition is caused by either permanent (chronic) or temporary (acute) damage to the brain. Some examples of chronic organic psychosis are lead poisoning, post traumatic head injury, post meningitic brain damage and multiple sclerosis. Acute organic psychoses are more frequently seen in drug intoxication due to prescription medications and illicit drugs such as amphetamines, PCP and LSD. Drug withdrawal syndromes such as delirium tremens as seen in alcoholics also produce organic psychoses.

## Management of the Psychotic Patient

The emergency management of the psychotic patient depends on the acuteness and severity of the condition, the type of psychotic illness, past psychiatric history, the presence of a suicidal or homicidal risk, and the availability of a social support system, i.e., family, friends, place to live, etc.

Assessment of these variables will provide valuable information that is used in developing a treatment plan for the patient. The comprehensive management of the patient will include interventions at several levels — the biological, pyschological and social strategies.

## Biological Therapy

Drug therapy for the acutely psychotic patient is usually the most important and immediate intervention. The choice of antipsychotic drug and the mode of administration is dependent on the following variables. Previous drug response history — patients generally respond better to the same drug or related compound. Allergic reactions and sensitivity to particular drugs are also indications that aid in choosing a particular drug. The level of psychomotor agitation provides the basis for choosing a sedating low potency low dose drug (haloperidol, fluphenazine, thiothixene). Rapid tranquilization procedures are an alternative method of handling the severly agitated, acutely psychotic in crisis. Several successive injections of a high potency antipsychotic are administered until a satisfactory level of sedation is achieved. (For example, haloperidol or fluphenazine HCL 5 mgs IM every 30 minutes.) Vital signs (pulse, BP, resp) are monitored regularly during and after this procedure. Low potency drugs such as chlorpromazine are not generally used because of the sedative and hypotensive side effects of these drugs. The patients' level of motivation for treatment is often directly related to the amount of denial and degree of insight about their illness. The route of administering medications will depend on the reliability of the patient, and their level of cooperativeness.

## Psychosocial Interventions

Psychotic patients are always approached in an empathic, concerned and nonjudgmental fashion. Therapists have to reach out in this manner in order to develop rapport and engage the patient who is unable to discern reality in any coherent way. Precipitating dynamic stressors are explored and psychological support is readily provided. In-depth, uncovering forms of psychotherapy are generally avoided during the acute phase of the illness. Therapists also try to understand family dynamics, and mobilize social support networks and linkages that are necessary when the patient is to be discharged or transferred from the emergency treatment service.

## CONCLUSION

The development and growth of emergency mental health services in the U.S. are briefly reviewed. Four types of frequently encountered mental health emergencies are presented as illustrations of presenting problems, assessment procedures and management strategies as they occur on an emergency treatment service. The importance of adequate facilities, a multidisciplinary treatment team approach and the identification and utilization of available social support networks were stressed. In conclusion, this general overview is presented so that care providers are able to recognize immediate dangers when treating the mentally ill patient in crisis.

## REFERENCES

1. Gerson S, Bassuk E: Psychiatric Emergencies: An Overview. American Journal of Psychiatry, 137:1, 1-11, 1980.

2. Barton GM: Emergency Psychiatry: The Outlook for the Future. Psychiatric Annals, 12:8, 807-813, 1982.

3. Bartolucci G, Drayer CS: An Overview of Crisis Intervention in the Emergency Rooms of General Hospitals. American Journal of Psychiatry, 130:953-960, 1973.

4. Hankoff LD, Mischon MT, Tomlinson KE, *et al.*: A Program of Crisis Intervention in the Emergency Medical Setting. American Journal of Psychiatry, 131:47-50, 1974.

5. Muller J, Chafetz M, Blane H: Acute Psychiatric Services in the General Hospital: III. Statistical Survey. American Journal of Psychiatry, October Supplement, 46-57, 1967.

6. Chafetz M: The Effect of a Psychiatric Emergency Service on Motivation for Psychiatric Treatment. Journal of Nervous Mental Disorders, 140: 442-448, 1965.

7. Freedman AM, Kaplan HI, Sadock BJ: Modern Synopsis of Comprehensive Textbook of Psychiatry II. Baltimore: Williams and Wilkins, 1976, pp. 870-874.

8. Salby AE, Lieb J, Tancredi LR: Handbook of Psychiatric Emergencies. New York: Medical Examination Publishing Co., Inc., 1975.

9. Rosenbaum CP, Beebe JE: Psychiatric Treatment — Crisis/Clinic/Consultation. New York: McGraw-Hill, 1975, p. 27.

10. Dubin WR, Stolberg R; Emergency Psychiatry for the House Officer. New York: SP Medical and Scientific Books, 1981, pp. 61-65.

11. Bell CC, Palmer J: Security Procedures in a Psychiatric Emergency Service. Journal of National Medical Association, 73(9):835-842, 1981.

12. Ruben HZ: Recognition and Management of the Dangerous Patient. Community Medicine, 44(12):770-773, 1980.

13. Fauman BS, Fauman MA: Emergency Psychiatry for the House Officer. Baltimore: Williams and Wilkins, 1981, p. 80.

# Chapter 9

BASIC PSYCHOTHERAPY AND COUNSELING SKILLS

RICHARD CARLSON, M.D.

Psychotherapy can be described as the treatment of the mind ("psyche") or, perhaps better, as one person listening to and offering some assistance to another person having psychological difficulties. It has probably been practiced in some form in all cultures, even in antiquity, because it is, in its simplest form, a basic mode of offering emotional help to a fellow human being. Counseling usually refers to guiding, directing, advising, and instructing people with an emphasis on problem–solving and generally deals with less serious psychopathology (1).

The formal study of psychotherapy goes back to about the middle of the last century, when physicians working in the field of neurology attempted to observe and analyze the workings of the mind (2). They noticed conscious and unconscious processes in their patients and there was a reproducibility of phenomena, from patient to patient, and in the same person. For instance, slips of the tongue occurred in people and these could be further analyzed as to their meanings. Also, grief or depression occurred regularly in people experiencing similar events, such as losses.

The earliest form of psychotherapy known as psychoanalysis is the one which usually comes to people's minds. This has major historical roots with Sigmund Freud and has contributed greatly to the understanding of dynamic psychological processes in general and to the development of many other forms of psychotherapy (3).

## BASIC PRINCIPLES OF PSYCHOTHERAPY

It may be helpful now to look at the five W's (what, why, who, when, and where) and the how of psychotherapy to better understand it in its basic applications (4).

As to the first question — *what* is psychotherapy? — we should look at basic human relationships and interactions for some understanding. It is, first of all, a treatment — a therapy — and, as such, implies that there is a problem in the mental or emotional functioning of a person. The therapy uses whatever conventional, established means are necessary to help the individual achieve a better state of adjustment within himself and the environment and to become less symptomatic. For example, a person who has always felt rather inadequate and lacking self-esteem and who begins feeling depressed could be helped in psychotherapy by examining the origins of this low self-esteem, his difficulty looking at positive aspects of himself, how these things affect his general mood and functioning in life, and how he could go about things more beneficially for himself.

In psychotherapy, one person (usually called the therapist) assists the other person (often referred to as the patient or client) to focus on his own inner psychological workings and relationships with others. Man is a social animal and, therefore, psychiatric symptoms usually are related to the functioning of the person in his environment.

We should also consider here what *is not* psychotherapy. Such recent and innovative developments as EST (Erhard Seminars Training), encounter groups, marathons, primal therapy and rebirthing should not be thought of as psychotherapy. Transactional analysis (T.A.), gestalt therapy, reality therapy, logotherapy, rational-emotive therapy and cognitive therapy are examples of techniques that developed from standard psychotherapies and are marginally related. Biofeedback, relaxation training and behavioral therapy are based on learning theories and represent very different kinds of treatment methods than psychotherapy.

The question of "what" now must lead to the important question of: *How* does psychotherapy work? This question relates as well to important human interrelationships. The therapeutic relationship itself involves two people. This is really the basis of the therapy — that one person is seen in a helping role and another person, suffering to some extent, turns to that person for aid. Empathy — the ability of someone to put himself in another's situation and to try to experience how it feels — is a basic key to the success of psychotherapy, or for any successful relationship for that matter. Empathy exists because all of us have common experiences. An example of empathy would be when one person relates the loss of a loved one, and the other person can feel some of what it feels like, because loss is a common tragic human experience. In therapy, the sharing of empathetic feelings is important, because it allows for ventilation, expression and acceptance of very significant emotions. Sympathy is counterproductive in therapy because both individuals experience the event to the same degree and one of them is not objective enough to remove himself from the problem and offer some strength to the other. An example of sympathy would be a patient telling a therapist about how difficult his boss is, and the therapist agreeing wholeheatedly while relating his own troubles with superiors.

The therapeutic encounter simulates in many ways some of our earlier important relationships. Anyone entering into treatment will experience this phenomenon with the therapist. It provides a basic setting in which insights into behaviors and in which growth can be achieved. This phenomenon is called transference (5). Specifically it refers to the unconscious feelings that an individual has or had toward another significant person, usually a parent, which are then transferred onto the therapist. This provides a setting in which to examine the development and important relationships of the person in the context of therapy. This is even stronger than empathetic feelings and serves as a powerful tool in the relationship developed in the treatment process, in that it assists the patient to examining himself and his psychodynamics.

During various types of psychotherapy, the therapist always attempts to help the person observe and analyze himself, to use healthier and more productive defense mechanisms, to deal with realities and to allow his ego strengths to be temporarily borrowed by the patient — all of these having the goal of alleviation of emotional distress and promotion of psychological growth.

*Why* does psychotherapy work? This has already been partially examined and really relates to the other questions that follow as well. Why is psychotherapy used as opposed to other treatments? It provides a close relationship over a period of time in which psychological functions of the person are examined. It takes time, and this is one drawback, but it is not easy for a person to examine such intangible and immeasurable things as thoughts and feelings. The setting of psychotherapy involving two people seems to promote this process however.

*Who* can do psychotherapy? Essentially anybody who is willing, interested in the patient, empathetic and has had some training in the principles and techniques of psychotherapy/counseling. Some research has shown that one of the most important factors in the success of psychotherapy is the therapist's interested, empathetic attitude (6). His skills, knowledge and artful use of psychotherapeutic techniques are important, but they probably only assist the therapist in his successful treatment. A caring, interested attitude is essential. This, of course, is true in any human relationship, and we see it repeated in the therapeutic encounter.

Jokes often center around bartenders or taxi drivers giving counseling to people in distress. These jokes highlight a truth, which is that these people, and many others, frequently do give support and allow a person to ventilate their problems. Psychotherapy, as we shall see, goes several steps further than that. Besides airing one's problems to a listener, the patient is confronted, allowed to observe his own behavior, to discover some hidden meanings in what he is doing and to make changes in his behavior.

The clergy, especially those trained in counseling, are particularly suited to helping people in distress. Individuals frequently turn toward their minister, priest or Rabbi in times of crisis and receive emotional, psychological and spiritual support. Often, they are referred later for further treatment by other mental health professionals.

The question of *when* in psychotherapy can be discussed from various aspects. As to time, people usually seek out help when a crisis is occurring or when they have symptoms which have become more pronounced or intolerable. From the therapist's point of view, psychotherapy is appropriate when the person is symptomatic, such as suffering from depression or anxiety, or is behaving in a maladaptive way, such as confronting authorities like his boss in a hostile manner with the possibility of losing his job. The person should be able to realize that his behavior is non-productive, should have some insight that he is having emotional difficulties, should want to change and should have strengths to be able to look into himself to gain further understanding to make changes. People with a moderate degree of mental retardation, those with marked antisocial personality disorders, those with active psychotic symptoms that put them out of touch with reality, and people with some brain damage, such as from trauma, alcohol, or a neurological disorder are usually not amenable to psychotherapy. If they are, they may receive only superficial help for some specific symptom. The above provides answers as to *where* and in what situations psychotherapy can be used.

## TYPES OF PSYCHOTHERAPY

We should now examine the various kinds of individual psychotherapies. Basically, these can be grouped into three types; psychoanalysis, psychoanalytically–oriented psychotherapy, and supportive psychotheraphy.

*Psychoanalysis* was developed by Sigmund Freud to treat patients by analyzing the unconscious aspects of their functioning and the effects of unconscious mechanisms on conscious behavior. This treatment is more appropriate for those who are symptomatic, such as with chronic anxiety or depression, and who are relatively well intact pyschologically to withstand the rigors of this intensive analysis.

Freud recommended the use of the couch to facilitate the analysis. Free associations, or the patient saying whatever comes to his mind, and dream analysis are tools used to help the patient examine his unconscious. Transference, and resistance to examining the unconscious, are very important processes in the analysis and they must be examined.

This is an intensive therapy that not everyone can tolerate. Sessions may be four or five times per week for an hour, the duration of treatment lasting a couple of years to perhaps eight or ten years in some cases.

Freud was able to examine sexual and aggressive features of childhood that occur normally. Difficulties in one or more of the phases of development may result in symptoms, brought on by unconscious turmoil. By analyzing and uncovering those thoughts and feelings, the patient could resolve them on a more conscious level.

This treatment approach requires special training and skills of the therapist, who has undergone personal analysis to allow him to have a better understanding of his own dynamic make-up.

*Psychoanalytically–oriented psychotherapy*, like classical psychoanalysis, may require several years, but usually is less intense. The couch is not used, and free association and dream analysis are employed less frequently and less intensely. The same dynamic principles are used but, as the title implies, this type of therapy is oriented towards psychoanalysis and does not copy it. Many patients are suitable for this type of therapy. Like psychoanalysis, it examines intrapsychic processes and is insight–oriented.

In order to contrast the two, and to help in contrasting them with other psychotherapies, the following examples are offered:

## An Example of Psychoanalysis

*Patient:* I'm not sure why this depressed feeling comes over me.
*Therapist:* It would help if you could tell me more.
*Patient:* Well, I seem to start feeling that way just when the weekend is almost over. Do you think it could be my job?
*Therapist:* It's interesting that you should relate it to going back to work. Please go on.
*Patient:* Every Monday morning I am sick to my stomach. I can't concentrate on my work in the morning and I wish I could just stay in bed and never have to go out!
*Therapist:* Like a child with no responsibilities.
*Patient:* I never considered that. I always hated my younger brother who stayed home when I went to school.

In this example, the burden is on the patient to explore himself and what is happening. The therapist acts as a tool in assisting him by listening, clarifying, confronting, interpreting and asking the patient to reflect on his behavior.

## An Example of Psychoanalytically–Oriented Psychotherapy

*Patient:* I'm not sure why this depressed feeling comes over me.
*Therapist:* Would you tell me more about it, like when it comes on and how long it lasts?
*Patient:* It usually comes at the end of every weekend and on Mondays.
*Therapist:* What does it feel like?
*Patient:* I can't concentrate, I feel sick to my stomach, I don't want to go to work, I shake all over and I can't sleep Sunday nights.

*Therapist:* It seems you have some difficulty facing your work and your responsibilities. Maybe you would like to be a child again for awhile.

In this case, the therapist is more active but basically uses the same techniques. The patient must still intensely examine his inner self.

A very important and useful form of therapy is *supportive psychotherapy*, which includes counseling. The name implies that psychological support is given to the patient to assist him in returning to an adequate level of functioning as quickly as possible. Sometimes the person is in an acute crisis, other times there may be ongoing problems that are creating symptoms, and sometimes this type of therapy is used over a long period of time to help to maintain a person at a certain functional level. The appointments may be weekly or less frequent, and the treatment may be as short as a few sessions or may go on for years. People with situational problems in life, such as a marital crisis, or schizophrenics who are stabilized but are facing some stresses on a day-to-day basis, may be helped. The point is that this form of therapy is suitable for almost anybody. Techniques of psychological support used by the therapist include: listening, allowing the patient to ventilate, empathetic caring, reassurance, advice and guidance.

## An Example of Supportive Therapy

*Patient:* I would like some help in trying to cope with my job. I can't stand it, but I need the money.
*Therapist:* I see your dilemma, one that so many people have difficulty with.
*Patient:* The last time I felt like this I just quit the job!
*Therapist:* I certainly wouldn't advise you to do that. Maybe we can look at the problem together.
*Patient:* I agree. I know I shouldn't quit, especially since jobs are so scarce.
*Therapist:* Not only that. It would be a giving-up approach instead of trying to tackle the problem. And you came here wanting to do something about it.

In this example, the therapist and patient are both very active in an ongoing discourse. Most people can benefit from this type of therapy and occasionally a person has to become involved in a more intensive therapy later to deal with the problem.

## SUMMARY

Psychotherapy is a useful form of treatment for individuals who have emotional or psychological problems which result in anxiety, depression or difficulties in interpersonal relationships. More specific disorders, such as phobias, compulsions, schizophrenia and other types of symptom-formation, may also be helped. Psychoanalysis, psychoanalytically-oriented psychotherapy and supportive psychotherapy are all effective, accepted forms of individual psychotherapy.

Although psychotherapy holds basic tenets, experience in practicing it helps to develop the art of therapy and one's own individual style. Anyone interested enough in helping others and in developing his abilities in the use of psychotherapeutic techniques will be successful as a therapist.

## REFERENCES

1. Wolberg LR: The Practice of Psychotherapy: 506 Questions and Answers. New York: Brunner/Mazel, 1982, pp. 158–159.

2. Breuer J and Freud S: Studies of Hysteria, In: Standard Edition of The Complete Psychological Works of Sigmund Freud, Vol. 2. London: Hogarth Press, 1955.

3. Jones E: The Life and Work of Sigmund Freud. New York: Basic Books, 1953.

4. Wolbert LR: The Technique of Psychotherapy, 3rd Ed. New York: Grune & Stratton, 1977.

5. Freud S: The Dynamics of Transference, In: Standard Edition of The Complete Psychological Works of Sigmund Freud, Vol. 12. London: Hogarth Press, 1958a.

6. Truax CB and Mitchell KM: Research on certain therapist interpersonal skills in relation to process and outcome, In: Bergin AE and Garfield SL (Eds.), Handbook of Psychotherapy and Behavior Change: An Empirical Analysis. New York: Wiley, 1971.

# Chapter 10

BEHAVIOR THERAPY: AN OVERVIEW
AND APPLICATION FOR SEXUAL DYSFUNCTION

RAMON A. LAVAL, Ph.D.
PONCE SANDLIN, M.D.

Members of the nursing and other allied health professions often constitute the first contact for individuals needing treatment for emotional, psychological, or behavioral problems. The increased awareness and sensitivity regarding mental health issues by these professionals has made it easier for the emotionally distressed individual to receive more appropriate services. Nurses and other allied health professionals will undoubtedly continue to interact with patients who, because of a variety of psychiatric and physical conditions, are in need of mental health services. Thus, an understanding of prevalent theories and systems of psychotherapy and psychopathology seems extremely relevant to the training of nurses and other allied health professionals. One of the most important developments in the area of assessment and treatment of psychological and behavioral problems within the last 30 years comes under the rubric of behavior therapy. The purpose of this chapter is to provide an overview of behavior therapy or behavior modification as it is also called, and to explore its application in the treatment of psychiatric disorders in general and sexual dysfunctions in particular.

## DEFINITION

Behavior therapy refers to the application of scientifically established *conditioning* (learning) principles and techniques to a wide of variety of psychiatric problems. In other words, behavior therapy is a set of rules and methods that help to change or modify certain behaviors. The main objectives in this regard are to help maintain, increase, or develop appropriate behaviors and to decrease or extinguish inappropriate or problematic behaviors. This is done with the aid of principles which are based on an area of psychology dealing with theories of learning, namely *classical conditioning* and *operant conditioning.*

## DEVELOPMENT OF BEHAVIOR THERAPY

Most of the foundations for behavior therapy were being developed during the first half of this century in both Russia and the United States (1). However, it was not until the 1950s that behavior therapy emerged as a systematic body of knowledge that could be applied to the understanding and treatment of psychiatric disorders (2). At that time, the prevailing thinking about mental health and mental care was largely psychoanalytic; thus, the new line of thinking embodied in behavior therapy was received with skepticism by some, and controversy and rejection by others.

But, why would there be so much controversy and such a clash between two types of therapy which, after all, were aiming for the same basic objective: to decrease psychological suffering? There are numerous reasons that help explain the mutual rejection that existed between psychoanalysis and behavior therapy. First, while for psychoanalysis the target of attention was "the mind" with its unconscious conflicts, motives and feelings, for behaviorism the target was behavior, namely, only responses or actions which could be clearly specified, observed and measured in some way. Also, while psychoanalysts viewed many psychiatric symptoms as manifestations of some intrapsychic conflict, behaviorists insisted that symptoms were really manifestations of how people had learned to cope with life stress. Since symptoms are learned and maintained in exactly the same way as normal behavior, behaviorists insisted that symptoms could be treated directly through the application of techniques based on principles of learning rather than directly by dealing with some presumed unconscious conflict. Thus, behavior therapy developed from within a context of great controversy, with research exploring its efficacy invading the literature and helping it become one of the most rapidly growing methods of therapy among mental health professionals.

At present, the term behavior is interpreted much more broadly than it was during the 1950s. Thus, besides referring to overt responding, it also includes emotions, feelings, thoughts, cognitive and symbolic processes which *can be clearly specified and measured.*

Today, behavior therapy is used to treat a variety of psychatric problems and dysfunctional behaviors including phobias, generalized (free floating) anxiety, obsessive–compulsive disorders, interpersonal problems, and sexual difficulties among others. Behavioral techniques have been effectively used with autistic children, mentally retarded individuals, psychotic as well as non-psychotic patients. Furthermore, behavioral programs have been developed to be implemented in a variety of settings such as the home, the school classroom, inpatient psychiatric wards, outpatient clinics, and even in industry and business settings.

Subsequent sections of this chapter will provide some examples of what behaviorists assume are the basic two types of learning: *classical* and *operant conditioning.*

## Classical Conditioning

Classical conditioning was discovered by a Russian physiologist, Dr. Ivan Pavlov (3), who after receiving his medical degree in 1883 immersed himself in physiological research dealing with the digestive process. His work in this area gained him world wide recognition as the recipient of the Nobel Prize in 1904. It should be noted that at first Dr. Pavlov, using dogs as subjects, was not really studying the way these animals learned and that the discovery of classical conditioning came out of difficulties and frustrations he was experiencing when conducting his physiological experiments.

Pavlov had a number of questions he wanted to answer such as what initiates secretion of gastric juices in the stomach when food was given to the dog. For this purpose, he performed a series of surgical procedures on the animal so that the stomach and esophagus were separated from each other. With these procedures, Pavlov was able to put food in the mouth of the dog without it ever reaching the stomach, or he could put food directly in the stomach without it having to go through the mouth and the esophagus. He was also able to measure the secretions from the salivary glands of the animal (salivation). Would the dog salivate after food was placed in his mouth or after it was directly placed in his stomach? Surprisingly, the dog would start salivating at the mere sight of Pavlov, even if he did not have any food with him. He also noted that if another person who had never fed the dog entered the laboratory, the animal wouldn't even blink. His experiments were completely ruined not once or twice, but many times in this fashion. Full of frustration, he completely rejected the notion that the dog was "thinking" about or imagining the food and thus engaging in "psychic secretion." Instead, he hypothesized that the dog *"learned"* or was *conditioned* to respond (salivate) at Pavlov's sight since repeatedly this experience was followed by his feeding the dog. Thus, according to Pavlov, he had produced an *acquired* or *conditioned* reflex in the animal.

Perhaps at this point it would be helpful to provide a description on how this type of conditioning or learning occurs in general. This may be done more easily with the use of a diagram and by explaining each aspect of it. In the case of Pavlov's experiment, he was dealing with an innate or unlearned reflex. That is, food in the mouth invariably elicits salivation; this is not a learned process. Thus, food in the mouth is an unlearned or *unconditioned stimulus* (US) which elicits a natural or *unconditioned response* (UR), salivation. This innate reflex is symbolized as follows:

$$\text{US} \longrightarrow \text{UR}$$
$$\text{(food in mouth)} \qquad \text{(salivation)}$$

Now, with respect to salivation, seeing the experimenter is in itself a completely neutral stimulus. In other words, seeing an experimenter does not naturally elicit salivation. However, the dog repeatedly experienced the following associations

$$\text{Dog saw Pavlov} \longrightarrow \text{Pavlov fed the dog} \longrightarrow \text{Dog salivated}$$

Seeing Pavlov and receiving food became associated one with the other, creating the following learned or conditioned reflex:

$$\text{Dog saw Pavlov} \longrightarrow \text{Dog salivated}$$

In other words, seeing the experimenter, in this case Pavlov, became a learned or *conditioned stimulus* (CS) which was now able to elicit salivation. And salivation had now become a learned or *conditioned response* (CR). We can symbolize this conditioned reflex in the following manner:

CS         ⟶         CR

(seeing Pavlov)          (salivation)

We have explained different aspects of the classical conditioning process. At this point we will provide a diagram illustrating how the entire process works with a description of how classical conditioning operates in general:

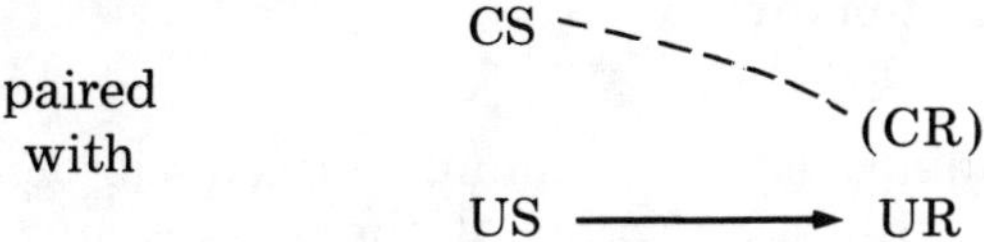


This implies that if you take any *neutral stimulus* and you pair it enough times with any *innate stimulus* (US), it is possible to get the *neutral stimulus* (CS) to elicit or bring about a response (CR) similar to the innate response (UR).

This type of learning takes place not only with dogs and other animals, but also with humans. Also, it applies to a great deal of important learning during infancy and childhood.

Perhaps the question arises of what classical conditioning has to do with emotional or psychological problems. It should be noted that there are a wide variety of innate reflexes that could be conditioned to any neutral stimuli. These innate reflexes can range from constriction of the pupil to light, to rapid heartbeat to electric shock, to a fear response when one is presented with a loud noise, to sexual arousal when stimulation of the genital area occurs. As was previously explained, any neutral stimulus may acquire the power to elicit a response very similar to the innate response. For example, a great variety of neutral stimuli can be conditioned to elicit a response very similar to the one observed in the case of sexual arousal to stimulation of the genital area. In fact, a number of fetishes or sexual arousal to objects such as shoes or underwear can be understood as having been developed through classical conditioning. This can be illustrated with the following diagrams:

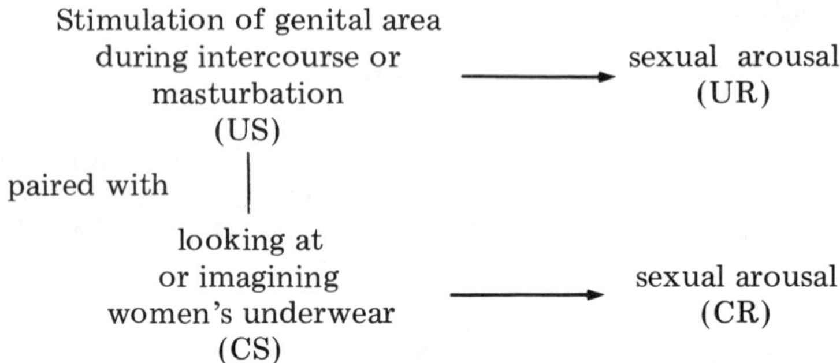


So, if looking at or imagining women's underwear is paired enough times with stimulation of the genital area, at one point looking at or imagining women's underwear (CS) will undoubtedly result in sexual arousal (CR). And, if this association becomes the main focus rather than a peripheral aspect of sexual activity, we could say without uncertainty that a *fetish* to women's underwear has been developed. A very important process which greatly extends the range of stimuli to which humans in particular can become conditioned to show fear, sexual excitement or other responses is that involved in *higher order conditioning*. It means that a previously neutral stimulus which has become a conditioned stimulus can serve to condition other neutral stimuli to elicit responses similar to the original, unconditioned one.

At this point, it is worth noting that behaviorists believe that virtually all phobias, that is persistent, irrational fears to a specific object, activity or situation, are simply classical conditioned fears of previously neutral objects. Perhaps this could become more clear after discussing the impact that another person had in the area of behavior therapy, the American psychologist, John B. Watson, who is considered to be the founder of behaviorism (4). Although Pavlov was the first behaviorist, Watson was the first one to use the term, and he soon became the leading figure of behaviorism. As a graduate student in psychology during the early 1900s, he was very argumentative and repudiated most of the theories about psychological functioning that were predominant during his time. He was very intolerant of such concepts as "mind" or "consciousness" used to describe human psychological functioning. For him, psychological functioning was no more than a series of behaviors and actions. According to him, emotions or feelings like love or hate were the result of changes in the muscles and the gland system. He insisted that "thinking" was merely the movement of vocal cords taking place while the individual engaged in sub-vocal (quiet) speech.

It was during the early 1900s that Watson first heard about classical conditioning, even before Pavlov's writings had been translated into English. Because of Watson's orientation and his repudiation of the writings in psychology at the time, the work of Pavlov made such overwhelming sense to him that he asserted that classical conditioning was the only form of learning and the basis for all of human functioning. Watson went even further in stating that all human behaviors were mere reflexes, a few of them innate, but, most of them learned or classically conditioned (5).

Behaviorists believe that phobias are irrational fears to specific objects, situations or animals which have been classically conditioned; that is, phobias are learned fears. Watson was the first and only person to experimentally develop a phobia in a child (6). Needless to say, by today's standards it would be considered unethical to attempt to do what Watson did in this famous experiment. The experiment is generally known as the case of Albert B.

Albert, an 11-month-old boy, enjoyed playing with furry animals and was so fearless that when presented with a white rat, he would happily reach for it. Watson decided to condition a phobia into this normal, fearless child and then to extinguish or de-condition it. In order to carry out his proposed plan, Watson placed a white rat in front of Albert, and just as the boy was eagerly trying to reach for it, Watson then struck a steel bar, making a very loud noise. This procedure was repeated a number of times until Albert soon had developed an intense fear of the animal. As the experiment continued, Watson realized that the child had not only developed a phobia for white rats, but he had also *learned* to be afraid of many furry things. Thus, little Albert also became very much afraid of a fur coat, of wool or cotton, and even of a Santa Claus mask. In other words, Albert showed *generalization* of a fear response to a variety of objects similar to the original one (white rat).

With this example of a classically conditioned fear in mind, consider how a conditioned fear might result in a different type of problem such as inhibited sexual excitement or what has also been termed frigidity or impotence. For this purpose, a summary of an actual clinical case is presented:

MV, a 24-year-old graduate student, came to a university clinic complaining of sexual difficulties. He appeared to have more than adequate social skills and was moderately attractive. He did not report, nor did he exhibit any serious psychopathology although his sexual problem had resulted in some mild feelings of depression and some heterosexual anxiety. MV defined his problem as a partial failure to maintain an erection during sexual intercourse, resulting in a frequent inability to complete the sexual act. He also indicated that he would generally wake up in the morning with a full erection and that he had never experienced problems with impotency while masturbating (information which seemed to contradict the presence of an organic basis to his presentation). MV further explained that he had been experiencing these difficulties for the last two years, during which time he had only been able to achieve a full erection and to complete the sexual act on five different occasions. Prior to that time, he appeared to have had a relatively normal dating as well as sexual life, with his first sexual experience occuring at age 18. During the assessment interview, MV provided the following information which helped determine from a behavioral viewpoint how his difficulties began. Approximately two years prior to his coming to the clinic, he was dating a female friend who was living at one of the college dorms. They had been seeing each other for about 4 months and had begun having sexual intercourse during the third month of their relationship. Since the friend lived in a dorm which exercised very rigid visiting regulations and at the same time she also shared a room with another student, their sexual relations always took place at his apartment. One evening, after having gone out for dinner, he suggested, as it had become the pattern, that they go to his place. She explained, however, that on this occasion she could not go as she was expecting an important telephone call from her parents early the next morning. Instead, she told him that her roommate was out of town at the time and would probably not return until the next day, so why didn't he stay with her at the dorm. Now, he was somewhat surprised as he was very much aware of the visiting regulations and had always feared the consequences of being caught entering, or leaving the dorm at the wrong time. With quite a bit of apprehension he nevertheless accepted the invitation. They somehow managed to get him into the room unnoticed, but as he recalled during the interview, once there, he was unable to relax and continued feeling apprehensive.

He explained that shortly after they had entered the room they began kissing and engaging in sexual foreplay, an experience which this time seemed not to be as gratifying as it had been in the past. A few minutes after they had begun having intercourse, they were suddenly interrupted by a loud continuous ringing bell; the sound of a fire alarm. They both jumped out of the bed not knowing what to do. He recalled having been extremely afraid. But then the bell stopped ringing, only to start again a few seconds later. It was at this point that she realized that this meant that this was a fire drill and that they were in no real danger. All she had to do, she explained to him, was to go down the stairs to the first floor and stay by one of the exits, check with the supervisor, and then return to her room.

For MV, this was the beginning of what would become approximately two years of sexual difficulties. The fear he had experienced had completely blocked whatever sexual arousal he had on that occasion. Later on, while he would not experience this same fear when engaging in sexual intercourse, he would nevertheless feel anxious, and this anxiety would block his arousal rendering him unable to maintain an erection. This case will provide the basis for the subsequent discussion of specific techniques of the behavioral treatment of sexual dysfunctions.

## Operant Conditioning

About the same time that Pavlov was establishing the principles of classical conditioning, Thorndike, a famous American psychologist was studying the process involved in a second form of learning (7). His contribution to the area of learning was organized under the rubric of the *law of effect*. He later referred to it as trial and error learning which subsequently became known as *instrumental conditioning*. It was during the late 1930s that another American man, Skinner, performed literally thousands of experiments, most of them with pigeons, and using Thorndike's Law of Effect as his guiding framework established the basic principles and technology of what he called *operant conditioning* (8). It should be noted that the concepts mentioned above: law of effect, trial and error learning, instrumental conditioning and operant conditioning, all refer to the basic learning process.

In discussing the classical conditioning process, nothing was mentioned about reinforcing or rewarding certain behaviors for the purpose of increasing, strengthening or maintaining these behaviors. In fact, the emphasis was in the appropriate pairing or association of certain stimuli which resulted in the learning of a conditional response. Also, it was not necessary for the animal or the individual to be motivated before he could learn. For example, Pavlov's dog did not need to be hungry in order to be conditioned to salivate. Furthermore, the animal or individual did not need to be actively trying to do anything: conditioning occurred mechanically. Despite the examples about classical conditioning provided in the previous section, there is a great amount of learning that cannot be delegated to this procedure alone, and a considerable number of behavioral problems can be understood as being learned through *operant conditioning*.

Operant conditioning emphasizes the importance of reinforcement during learning. But in order for reinforcement to occur, the individual needs to respond or *operate* upon the environment. Thus, whereas in classical conditioning the responses were reflexive or involuntary, in operant conditioning the responses are *voluntary* ones. Furthermore, level of motivation plays a very important role in this type of learning. For instance, to teach a dog to bring the newspaper every morning, one could not use food as a reinforcer if the animal was satiated at the time; the dog needs to be motivated; that is, the dog needs to be at least a little bit hungry.

The principles involved in operant conditioning are somewhat more elaborate and technical than those in classical conditioning. Thus, to simplify matters, a description of how a very basic operant conditioning experiment would be conducted is in order. To conduct his controlled studies, Skinner developed an instrument which is generally known as a Skinner box. This is a box large enough to hold the animal being studied, usually a pigeon or a rat. Inside the box there is a key or a lever that, if pushed, delivers a pellet of food. When first placed in the box, animals usually perform a number of movements or operations such as touching or sniffing parts of the cage or climbing the walls. Finally, the animal pushes the lever and a pellet of food is delivered. Eventually, the animal's main operation inside the box is to press the lever and to eat the food being delivered. At this point, the animal has become the subject of operant conditioning and has learned to press the bar for reinforcement. Now, the following definition will help put this example into a more general perspective so that the learning of other types of behaviors can also be understood. Operant conditioning refers to a process in which the frequency of occurrence of a behavior is modified or controlled by its consequences. Here, the concepts of reinforcement and punishment are very important, and they are always defined in terms of the effects on behavior. The word *reinforce* implies that a behavior is strengthened or increased, whereas the word *punish* connotes that a behavior is weakened or decreased. There are basically two types of reinforcers: positive and negative.

A *positive reinforcer* is really a reward, or something given to an organism or an individual after a desirable action; for example, giving a child candy or letting him watch TV after he has completed his homework. If, in the future, the child increases the frequncy of this studying behavior in order to be reinforced as he was before, *positive reinforcement* is taking place. One could also *negatively reinforce* the child in order for him to increase his studying behavior by yelling and screaming at him *until* he starts studying. In other words, a *negative reinforcer* is a stimulus (screaming and yelling) which, when removed (stop screaming) immediately following the occurrence of a behavior (child starts studying), increases the likelihood of that behavior recurring.

An example will help to understand further how these two types of reinforcement operate. Little Peter is a 3–year–old boy who will not go to sleep at night unless his parents accompany him to his room, get him in bed and then read stories for him. The problem is that this process sometimes takes hours, and if his parents leave the room before little Peter is asleep, the boy starts crying and throws a temper tantrum until the parents return to the room. In this situation, both positive and negative reinforcement are taking place concurrently. The parents' returning to the room and reading him stories is a positive reinforcer which increases the likelihood that little Peter will cry again the next night. At the same time, the parents' behavior — returning to the room — is being negatively reinforced. The negative reinforcer here is the boy's crying behavior which is stopped after the parents return to the room, thus increasing the likelihood that the parents will repeat this behavior the following night when little Peter cries again.

The question arises whether or not one learns behavior, actions, or responses only if he is reinforced every time he does them. One could cite thousands of things individuals have done which were not followed by a reinforcer, yet continued doing them again and again. The concept of reinforcement schedule is important in this regard. There are two general schedules of reinforcement, fixed and variable. A *fixed schedule* is one in which reinforcement occurs after a certain fixed number of responses or after a fixed period of time. For example, a worker may get paid $10 after he has manufactured 1,000 belts (*fixed ratio*), or a worker may get paid every 4 weeks (*fixed interval*). Another typical example of a fixed interval schedule of reinforcement can be seen when a professor gives an exam every 2 weeks. Student response right after a test is very low or infrequent (students do not study as they know they will not be tested for a while). One week after the test, students become a little nervous; so they carry the textbook with them everywhere they go, but they still do not study. The night before the test, almost everybody is responding very intensely (cramming) because the next morning the professor will reinforce the students by giving them a test.

A *variable schedule* is one in which reinforcement occurs irregularly, but on the average, after a fixed number of responses (*variable ratio*) or a fixed period of time (*variable interval*). Variable schedules produce the highest rate of responding, and these responders are very hard to extinguish even after reinforcement has been completely stopped. A good example of a *variable ratio schedule* of reinforcement involves the operation of slot machines in casinos. Assume that one can hit the jackpot every 50 plays *on the average*. Sometimes it may happen after pressing the lever once or sometimes after pressing it 100 times. Thus, the more quarters one puts in, the more jackpots he will hit. However, the more he plays, the more money he loses, but the occasional jackpot has more reinforcing value than the numerous losses experienced. In the case of the *variable interval schedule*, imagine the professor who instead of always giving a test every 2 weeks, gives them so that they will, on the average, be every two weeks. Sometimes one week may separate the tests and other times three weeks. Under these circumstances, the typical student will learn that if he just studies regularly, he will alwyas be prepared for the tests.

An organism can be taught to learn almost anything that it is physically capable of doing, simply by careful management of consequences. However, if every time one wants to teach someone to learn something he has to wait first for that behavior to occur so that is can be reinforced, he may have to wait forever. Skinner, for example, wondered about the following: Is a pigeon physically able to play ping-pong? Nothing about the pigeon's anatomy would impede its being able to hold a miniature paddle in its beak and hit a ball over a net. If one waits for a pigeon to do just that in order to reinforce that behavior, thus increasing the likelihood that his behavior will recur, he will probably wait forever. Instead, Skinner decided to systematically reinforce successive approximations to the ultimate desired behavior: "Playing ping-pong." Thus, using operant conditioning principles, he would first reinforce the pigeon every time it walked toward the paddle, then every time the pigeon moved the beak toward the paddle, next only when it touched the paddle, then only when it picked it up, etc., until the pigeon was reinforced only for hitting a ball over a net with a paddle. He taught a second pigeon to do the same, and he finally had two very unusual ping-pong players. This procedure of conditioning a behavior not currently in the organisms's behavioral repertoire by reinforcing closer and closer approximations of the desired behavior, resulting eventually in the acquisition of that behavior is called *shaping*.

## BEHAVIOR THERAPY: TECHNIQUES AND APPLICATIONS

It is not possible to talk about behavior therapy as representing one coherent and systematic method of doing therapy. Instead behavior therapy includes a number of techniques that can be applied depending on the type pf problem that one wishes to modify and on the individual exhibiting that problem. However, what unifies all of these different techniques which form the armamentarium of behavior therapy is the emphasis in classical and operant conditioning. These two forms of learning were discussed in previous sections. Most behavior therapists adhere to a three-factor theory of learning. Thus, in addition to emphasizing classical and operant conditioning, they also underline the importance of a third type of learning, *cognitive conditioning*. In so doing, they acknowledge the central and paramount role that the individual's internal, cognitive life plays in any type of learning. It is not sufficient to know how environmental stimuli and consequences affect a person's behavior, but it is also necessary to assess how that person understands, labels, construes, and perceives his own behavior and the environment. This cognitive life is represented in different opinions, feelings, thoughts or even symbolic manifestations that the individual has about himself and his environment.

Some of the most commonly used techniques that behavior therapists use when treating psychiatric or behavior problems will now be summarized.

## Systematic Desensitization

This technique developed by a South African psychiatrist, Joseph Wolpe (9), is aimed specifically at the reduction and alleviation of maladaptive anxiety. It basically follows the principle of *counter conditioning*. In other words in systematic desensitization one tries to substitute an emotional response which is inappropriate or maladaptive to a given situation (anxiety) by one that is appropriate or adaptive (relaxation). This method has been shown to be very effective in treating anxiety reactions conditioned to specific situations or events. It has also been used to treat a variety of other disorders which are not obviously phobic in nature such as impotency, insomnia, and alcoholism.

In the clinical case involving MV provided in a preceding section, systematic desensitization (SD) was used to treat his sexual impotency. A number of steps are taken before one decides to use SD. First, one has to determine whether anxiety or fear plays an important role in the patient's problem. Second, it is also necessary to assess whether the problem is associated with irrational anxiety. For example, the anxiety is considered irrational if there is evidence that the patient has sufficient skills (social, sexual, etc.) for coping with whatever it is he fears. If the fear is in some way rational either because the patient is lacking in some pertinent skills or because the situation about which the patient is afraid is in fact dangerous, SD may be contraindicated. For instance, one would not want to desensitize a patient who complains of extreme anxiety while driving under the influence of alcohol. Next, one also needs to determine whether desensitization can be done in the therapist's office or "in-vivo" in the natural setting.

Three different procedures are involved in SD. The first one involves training the patient in deep relaxation techniques. The second one involves the development of a hierarchy of events associated with the patient's fears. During the final stage of SD, the patient is asked to imagine the events described in the hierarchy while in a state of relaxation. After considering these and other factors, it was decided that SD would be used to treat MV's impotency.

A very effective method for inducing a deep state of muscle relaxation involves the successive tensing and relaxing of voluntary muscles in an orderly sequence until all of the main muscle groups of the body are relaxed. Relaxation training may take approximately three to four 40-minute sessions. During this time the hierarchy of relevant events is also developed.

The hierarchy is a graduated series of situations or scenes that the patient is asked to imagine while in a state of relaxation. The scenes consist of realistic, concrete situations relevant to the patient's fears. The complete hierarchy is to be graduated in terms of the degree of anxiety elicited by the different scenes, and in most cases ten items are sufficient to form a hierarchy. The patient is asked to rate each item on a 10 point anxiety scale. As an example, the following items with their correspondent level of anxiety were included in MV's hierarchy.

| *Items* | *Anxiety Score* |
|---|:---:|
| Being alone at a public place with an attractive woman | 1 |
| Being alone at his or her apartment with an attractive woman | 4 |
| Kissing and caressing a woman while both are completely dressed | 8 |
| Both completely undressed and ready to have intercourse | 10 |

After the patient has been trained in deep muscle relaxation and the hierarchy has been developed, the final stage of SD begins. The patient is comfortably seated in a chair (he may be asked to lie down on a couch) and asked to relax. After the patient achieves a good level of relaxation, the therapist describes the first scene to be imagined — the item with the lowest anxiety score. When the patient signals a clear image, the therapist allows approximately 7 seconds to elapse after which the patient stops imagining that scene. If the patient signals anxiety during the presentation, he is asked to stop imagining the scene and to return to a state of relaxation. After 15–20 seconds, the patient should be ready for the second presentation of the same scene. Before introducing the next hierarchy item the same procedure is repeated.

A typical SD session lasts from 15 to 40 minutes depending on the patient's ability to concentrate. A patient undergoing SD is strongly recommended not to place himself in a situation corresponding to a hierarchy item not yet desensitized. Length of therapy may range from one to twenty sessions. For example, MV was able to have intercourse without difficulties after 9 SD sessions.

## Flooding (Implosive Therapy)

Unlike SD which relies on relaxation to substitute the anxiety experienced by different graduated items, flooding involves prolonged exposure to high intensity anxiety–producing situations, without relying on relaxation. Flooding, which may be conducted in–vivo or imaginally, assumes that anxiety and other fears are maintained because the anxious individual will tend to avoid or escape the source of his apprehension (e.g., open places, snakes, driving, sexual relations), and thus, extinction of the fears will never take place. A therapist using flooding with an individual suffering from a fear or driving may provide the patient with the following scene to be imagined: he is driving his car, and he is terribly nervous. He suddenly realizes that he is so anxious that he becomes nauseated. He then realizes he has lost control of his car and that he will probably have a terrible wreck . . . etc.

## Thought Stopping

This technique, aimed at decreasing obsessive thinking, uses a simple classical conditioning procedure. The patient is asked to verbalize his intrusive, obsessive thoughts. While the patient is in the process of verbalizing these thoughts, the therapist suddenly yells *STOP*. This procedure is repeated a number of times in a systematic manner. Later, the patient is asked not to verbalize, but to merely think about his obsessions and to signal the therapist when this is occurring. Again, the therapist yells *STOP*. Finally, the patient is asked to both think of the obsession and to imagine *STOP* in his mind. Eventually, the patient ceases obsessing.

## Cognitive Conditioning

This type of therapy is based on the assumption that the way a patient thinks about, or construes or labels his experiences, will result at times in strong maladaptive emotional reactions such as anxiety or depression. Albert Ellis, for example, insists that individuals become neurotic because they have a large number of irrational attitudes or propositions which guide their life (10). Some of these irrational thoughts include:

"—The idea that it is a dire necessity for an adult human being to be loved or approved by virutally every significant other person in his community.

—The idea that one should be thoroughly competent, adequate, and achieving in all possible respects if one is to consider oneself worthwhile.

—The idea that there is invariably a right, precise, and perfect solution to human problems and that it is catastrophic if this correct solution is not found."

There are four basic steps in this type of therapy. The first step involves the process of explaining to the patient that many of his emotions and feelings are the result of distressing statements he tells himself about a situation or event rather than being the result of the situation itself. During the second step, the therapist helps the patient identify some of these self-statements. In the third step, it is necessary to convince the patient of the irrational and self-defeating nature of these self-statements. Finally, the therapist models and reinforces alternative, more appropriate and constructive self-verbalizations which are incompatible with anxiety, depression or other maladaptive emotions.

## Biofeedback

The assumption here, is that if internal responses associated with different emotional states (e.g., heartrate, respiration rate, muscle tension, brain waves, etc.) are made external and can be visualized by using a monitor, the patient can be reinforced to produce changes in these responses. This technique has been used in many areas of medicine, and its usefulness continues to be evaluated.

## Token Reinforcement Programs

The token economy is an excellent example of how operant conditioning principles can be used to structure a relatively large setting or environment in order to help a large number of individuals. These programs have been used in a variety of settings ranging from the home to inpatient psychiatric wards.

The development of a token economy program involves a number of steps. First, a comprehensive list of behaviors (target behaviors) considered to be adaptive and appropriate for the patients or individuals involved is developed. In the case of a program to be implemented in a psychiatric ward, these behaviors may include a variety of basic personal and social skills, attending therapy sessions, participation at different meetings, engaging in appropriate speech, etc. Next, it is necessary to establish what will constitute the "backup reinforcers." These are the particular rewards (e.g., food, weekend pass, attending special activities, etc.) that token reinforcers can be exchanged for. One also needs to decide what type of tokens, representing the backup reinforcers, he will use. They may include different colored poker chips representing different values, points or check marks. Finally, one needs to establish the rules of exchange specifying the different value (in tokens) of different target behaviors and the number of tokens required to obtain various backup reinforcers.

## Other Techniques

A variety of other techniques are used to modify numerous maladaptive behaviors. Aversive counter-conditioning has been used to treat alcoholism, smoking and sexual deviations. Simple reinforcement procedures have been shown to be very effective in child management at the school and the home setting. Shaping techniques have been used to teach the autistic child to talk and the mentally retarded to add and subtract. Communications training has been quite effective in teaching partners to become more reinforcing to each other. Modeling and role-playing have been very useful in teaching depressed, passive individuals to become happier and more assertive. These are only a few examples of different behavioral interventions and the behaviors they help modify.

## CONCLUSION

The purpose of this chapter was to discuss behavior therapy, its development, and its application in the treatment of psychiatric disorders, with particular attention paid to the treatment of sexual dysfunctions.

During the 1950s, behavior therapy was not very well received; it soon became an alternative approach to the treatment of behavioral problems. The foundations for this type of treatment and how it was being developed during the early 1900s in both Russia and the United States was also discussed as was the importance of classical and operant conditioning in this respect. Further discussion indicated that most behavior therapists adhere to a three-factor theory of learning. In this context, the importance of a third type of learning, cognitive conditioning, was emphasized.

Finally, the fact was noted that it is difficult to talk about behavior therapy as consisting of one coherent method of doing therapy. Instead, a number of techniques that come under the rubric of behavior therapy as they all emphasize the importance of learning theory in the treatment of behavioral problems were presented.

## REFERENCES


1. Turner SM, Calhoun KS and Adams HE (Eds.): Handbook of Clinical Behavior Therapy. New York: John Wiley & Sons, 1981, pp. 2-4.

2. O'Leary KD and Wilson GT: Behavior Therapy: Application and Outcome. New Jersey, Prentice-Hall, 1975, pp. 3-7.

3. Pavlov I: Conditioned Reflexes. New York: Oxford University Press, 1927.

4. Schultz DP: A History of Modern Psychology. New York: Academic Press, 1969.

5. Watson JB: Behaviorism. New York: Norton, 1930.

6. Watson JB and Rayner R: Conditioned emotional responses. J Experimental Psychology, 3:1-14, 1920.

7.  Thorndike EL: Human Learning, New York: Appleton, 1938.

8.  Skinner BF: The Behavior of Organisms. New York: Appleton, 1938.

9.  Wolpe J: Psychotherapy of Reciprocal Inhibition. Stanford: Stanford University Press, 1958.

10. Ellis A: Reason and Emotion in Psychotherapy. New York: Lyle Stuart, 1962.

# Chapter 11

## PHARMACOTHERAPEUTICS

OCTAVIO C. PINELL, M.D.
GEORGE L. ADAMS, M.D.

Since antiquity, physicians have attempted to modify behavioral problems using medicinal or chemical methods. The new psychopharmacological era, however, started at the mid part of the twentieth century when Cade (1) in Australia introduced lithium as an anti–manic drug. This event was closely followed duing the early 1950s by Delay and Deniker's discovery of the tranquilizing effect of chlorpromazine. Since then, many pharmacotherapeutic drugs have been introduced to treat other psychiatric disorders. Among the drugs most frequently prescribed for behavioral problems currently are the: 1) neuroleptics, 2) antidepressants, 3) anxiolytic sedatives, 4) psychostimulants, and 5) anti–manics. The authors will focus on providing a brief description of the psychotropic drugs in each of the above five groups, delineating their usefulness in the treatment of mentally ill, and their additional potential use outside of the field of psychiatry.

## NEUROLEPTICS

The neuroleptics are a group of compounds proven to be effective in the management of a broad range of psychotic symptoms and considered to be particularly useful in the management of schizophrenia and mania. The term neuroleptic refers to agents that:

1. have beneficial effects in disturbances of perception (hallucinations and illusions) and thinking (characteristic of psychosis) (2);
2. Reduce the duration of some psychotic disorders (3);
3. Long term neuroleptic medication administered to patients reduced the risk of relapse (3);
4. Moderate anxiety and psychomotor agitation (4);

5. Achieve their effects at doses far lower than those required to produce sleep (5);
6. Cause little dampening of the arousal response to afferent stimuli (6);
7. Do not produce a substantial degree of tolerance, physical dependence, or craving (7);
8. Lower the convulsive threshold (8); and
9. Produce extrapyramidal manifestations.

Neuroleptics have also been called major tranquilizers, antipsychotics, ataraxics, and neuroplegics. Yet the term neuroleptics is preferred because these drugs lead to various symptoms in humans which are characterized as the "neuroleptic syndrome," or neurologic syndrome. This syndrome comprises symptoms of psychomotor inhibition, modifying neurovegetative changes, disturbances in tonus, occasional extrapyramidal effects, and reduction in psychotic manifestations.

Moreover, the epithet "major tranquilizer" does not represent accurately the action of this psychopharmacologic class of agents. The term "antipsychotic" is not correct as some psychoses do not respond to these drugs. The name ataraxic, which means peace of mind, is not adequate because some patients become very concerned with some of the side effects, and the term neurologic is inaccurate because it implies paralyzing effect (9, 10).

## Classification of the Neuroleptics

The neuroleptics used presently in the U.S.A. could be classified into four groups according to their chemical structure:
1. The tricyclic neuroleptics (including the phenothiazines, the thioxanthenes, and the dibenzo–oxazepine derivatives);
2. The butyrophenone derivatives;
3. The rauwolfia alkaloids, benzoquinolizine, and various indole derivatives; and
4. Unclassified neuroleptics.

### Tricyclic Neuroleptics

*Phenothiazines:* The term phenothiazine refers to those agents containing a tricyclic nucleus of two benzene rings (pheno), joined through a central ring containing a sulphur atom (thio) and a nitrogen atom (azo), to which is attached a carbon side chain terminating in either a tertiary amine or a cyclic structure analogue of a tertiary amine. According to their chemical composition they may be divided into:

1. The aliphatic group, characterized by a three carbon straight chain;
2. The piperidine group characterized by a piperidine ring in the side chain;
3. The piperazine group characterized by a piperazine ring in the side chain.

*Thioxanthenes:* This category comprises tricyclics in which the nitrogen atom has been replaced by a carbon atom but leaving the sulfur atom. This type of molecule is a sulfur–containing (thio) structural analogue of xanthene. The thioxanthenes currently on the market have molecules with side chains of the aliphatic type (e.g., chlorprothixenes).

*Dibenzoxazepine derivatives:* These are tricyclic compounds with a piperazine ring and a centrally assymetrical ring.

## Butyrophenones

These are derivatives also called phenylbutyl piperidines that were synthesized from substances which are chemically related to pethidine (meperidine). The only butyrophenone routinely prescribed in the U.S.A. as an antipsychotic is haloperidol (Haldol®). Droperidol (Inapsine®) is an antipsychotic but is only available as an anesthetic at present.

## The Indole Derivatives

These compounds contain an indolic molecular structure.

## Rauwolfia Alkaloids

At the present time, the rauwolfia alkaloids have only a historical interest from the psychiatric aspect.

## Clinical Pharmacology

The phenothiazines, and in a similar fashion other neuroleptics, have the tendency to: 1) produce sedation; 2) block conditioned avoidance behavior; 3) have antimentic, antipruritic, and analgesic effects; 4) alter temperature regulation (phenothiazines produce poikilothermia) and skeletal muscle tone; 5) facilitate seizure discharge; 6) induce endocrine changes, including decreasing levels of growth hormone and increase prolactin release by the pituitary; 7) produce strong adrenergic and weaker peripheral cholinergic blocking; 8) induce local anesthesia (mainly tricyclic); 9) potentiate the action of different number of drugs; and 10) depress or stimulate the reticular activating system depending on dosage. In therapeutic doses for psychosis, the aliphatic and the piperidine side chains have more of a sedative action and marked negative side effects, such as orthostatic hypotension. The piperazine group produces more extrapyramidal manifestations (4).

## Mechanism of Action from the Psychiatric Aspect

Hypothetically speaking, it is believed that the antipsychotic effects of the neuroleptic drugs are associated with their ability to block dopaminergic transmission in the limbic system. Their potency in this respect is correlated with their clinical efficacy in schizophrenias (11); but they also show antidopaminergic activities in the striatum, hypothalamus, and reticular activating system (12, 13, 14).

## Dosages

In general, it could be said that the aliphatic and piperidine groups should be prescribed in hundreds of milligrams when treating psychosis (chlorpromazine, thioridazine and mesoridazine from 100 mg to 800 mg or more with chlorpromazine), whereas the piperazine group (trifluoperazine, perphenazine, prochlorperazine, fluphenazine, etc., should be prescribed in tens of milligrams — from 2 to 100 mg). In therapeutic doses for some psychosis, the aliphatic and the piperadine groups have a more accentuated anticholinergic and antiadrenergic action. The piperazine group has a more obvious antidopaminergic activity (4).

## Adverse Effects

Adverse effects related to neuroleptics could be classified as:
1. *Hypersensitivity reactions:* Characteristically, these occur during the first few days or first two or three months of treatment, are not related to drug dosage, are sometimes associated with

**CHEMICAL CLASSES AND DOSAGE RELATIONSHIP
AMONG ANTIPSYCHOTICS**

| *Drug and Class* | *Relative Potency in mg* |
| --- | --- |
| Phenothiazines | |
| Aliphatic | |
| Chlorpromazine | 100 |
| Piperidine | |
| Thioridazine | 100 |
| Mesoridazine | 50 |
| Piperacetazine | 10 |
| Piperazine | |
| Prochlorperazine | 15 |
| Perphenazine | 10 |
| Trifluoperazine | 5 |
| Fluphenazine | 2 |
| Thioxanthenes | |
| Thiothixene | 5 |
| Chlorprothixene | 100 |
| Butyrophenones | |
| Haloperidol | 2 |
| Dibenzoxazepines | |
| Loxapine | 10 |
| Indolics | |
| Molidone | 10 |

other manifestations of hypersensitivity, and positive challenge response may occur for years after the original action subsides. The two main hypersensitivity reactions are cholostatic jaundice, and skin reactions, generalized or localized, e.g., urticaria, maculopapular rashes, petechiae, edema, exaggerated tanning, exaggerated sunburn, excrematous lesions (9).

2. *Toxic effects:* Toxic effects are generally exaggerations of the pharmacological effects and increase in incidence and severity with increased dosage. Among the toxic effects which may be clinically detected are: 1) drowsiness (that is inversely related to the therapeutic effect); 2) extrapyramidal effects (perhaps the most frequent side effects of neuroleptic drugs) (15). Among the most frequent extrapyramidal effects are: 1) Dystonias, also called hyperkinetic-dystonic crises or excitomotor syndrome. They manifest themselves by sudden intermittent, but often persistent

spasms of individual muscle groups, particularly those of the neck, lips, tongue and eyes (e.g., involuntary protrusion of the tongue, mandibular spasms, torticollis, retrocollis, oculogyric crisis, torsion spasms, opisthotonos, all of which may be accompanied by perspiration, fever and pallor). They appear early in the treatment (from a few minutes to three days after the beginning of the neuroleptic therapy). 2) Akathisia, a motor unrest which manifests itself mostly in the legs; in mild cases patients tend to shuffle, whereas in more severe cases, patients are in constant motion, hardly able to sit still or lie down. This reaction usually appears within the first two weeks after the onset of treatment. 3) Drug induced parkinsonism, characterized by muscular rigidity, hypokinesia, mask like face, pill rolling tremor, waxy skin, excessive salivation, micrographia, monotonous and expressionless voice. This is usually fully developed in a period of three weeks. 4) Hypokinesia which is characterized by the slowing down of motor activity with fixed posture. It is usually noticed after 10 days; and 5) the rare rabbit syndrome (perioral movements that mimic the chewing movements of a rabbit) (9). Synthetic estrogenic hormones and hypoparathyroidism facilitate the appearance of these reactions; genetic factors may also contribute to EPM (16, 17).

It has been assumed that inhibition of transmission in DA neurons of the nigrostriatal systems and excessive activity of ACh are the main causes for these types of extrapyramidal manifesta-

| EXTRAPYRAMIDAL MANIFESTATIONS | |
|---|---|
| *Extrapyramidal Symptoms* | *Clinical Manifestations* |
| Dystonia | Sudden intermittent or persistent spasms of individual muscles, particularly those in the neck, lips, tongue and eyes. |
| Akathisia | Motor unrest, sometimes the patients are in constant motion. |
| Drug induced Parkinsonism | Muscular rigidity, hypokinesia, mask-like face, pill rolling tremor, waxy skin, excessive salivation, micrographia, monotonous and expressionless voice. |
| Hypohinesia | Slowing down in motor activity. |
| Rabbit Syndrome | Oral movements that mimic the chewing movements of a rabbit. |

tions (18). They can be treated with anticholinergic drugs like benztropine mesylate (Cogentin® 1-2 mg tid or qid); trihexyphenidyl (Artane® or Tremin® 2-5 mg tid or qid); biperiden (Akineton® 1-2 mg tid or qid); procyclidine (Kemadrin® 2.5-5 mg tid or qid). The use of amantadine, a dopamine releasing agent, in a dose of 50 to 100 mg tid or qid may be useful to control early extrapyramidal symptoms (19, 20). Mild cases can be handled by close reduction; at this time, prophylactic use of antiparkinsonia drugs is not advisable.

3. *Vegetative side effects:* They are most frequent in the beginning of treatment. Later on, there is an adjustment to them and the organism goes back to a vegetative equilibrium. They are related to anticholinergic or antiadrenergic manifestations. The outcome is often manifold and contradictory. Among these manifestations we find: hypotension, but occasionally hypertension, tachycardia, palpitations, hypersalivation or dryness of the mouth, diarrhea or constipation, fever or hypothermia, perspiration or anhidrosis, hot flashes or chills, pallor or reddening of the skin, sleepiness or insomnia, polyuria or urinary retention, bulimia or loss of appetite, hyperperistalsis or intestinal atonia, miosis or mydriasis, nausea and vomiting, delayed ejaculation or impotence (9).

4. *Catatonic reaction:* Severe akinetic, catatonic reaction and mutism have been associated with high doses of potent neuroleptics. Antiparkinsonia drugs may be of value in controlling these

---

**DRUGS USED TO TREAT  
EARLY EXTRAPYRAMIDAL MANIFESTATIONS**

| *Generic Name & Trade Name* | *Manufacturer* | *Typical Individual Dose for Adults* |
|---|---|---|
| Anticholinergic Drugs | | |
| Benztropine (Cogentin®) | Merck | 1-2 mg tid or qid |
| Trihexyphenidyl (Artane®) | Lederle | 2-5 mg tid or qid |
| (Tremin®) | Schering | 2-5 mg tid or qid |
| Biperiden (Akineton®) | Knoll | 1-2 mg tid or qid |
| Procyclidine (Kemadrin®) | Burroughs | 2.5-5 mg tid or qid |
| Diphenhydramine (Benadryl®) | Parke-Davis | 25-50 mg tid or qid |
| Dopaminergic Stimulant Drugs | | |
| Amantadine (Symmetrel®) | Endo Pharm. | 100-mg tid or qid |

manifestations, but improvement usually follows reducing the dosage.

5. *Withdrawal dyskinesia:* Another infrequent reaction is "withdrawal Dyskinesia" usually associated with rapid discontinuation of large doses of potent antipsychotic agents after withdrawing patients taking megadoses of haloperidol, trifluoperazine, or fluphenazine we may see as a complication an acute choreitcathetoic reaction, similar in appearance to tardive dyskinesia but lasting usually only a few days (21). Similar reactions have been described after abrupt discontinuation of the usual doses of antipsychotic agents in children and young adults.

6. *Biochemical side effects:* Increased alpha globulins (at the beginning of the treatment) which later on disappear. It may be accompanied by increased sedimentation rate (9).

7. *Hemopoietic system:* At the beginning of the treatment, we may see: transitory eosinophilia and short–lasting leucopenia and eosinopenia. Long term therapy may produce relative lymphocytosis and monocytosis. Agranulocytosis may appear in from 0.001 to 0.002% of the cases, most frequently found when taking more than 100 mg of the drugs. Usually, it appears during the first ten weeks of treatment. Anemias, thrombocytopenias and pancytopenias have been reported (9).

8. *Psychiatric side effects:* Among the most common psychiatric side effects are: 1) apathy, 2) somnolence, 3) sopor and comatose states, 4) insomnia, 5) delirium, 6) depression, and 7) depersonalization (22, 23, 24).

9. *Adverse effects* following long term use of antipsychotics. Long term treatment with antipsychotic drugs may produce: 1) pigmentary changes of skin and eyes (in the skin you may see violet hued decoloration in sunlight exposed areas of the skin; in the eyes you may detect whitish pearled formations or yellow brown deposits in lens, cornea and conjunctiva (25); pigment accumulation in the retina has been described in patients taking large doses of thioridazine (26); 2) hepatic changes (cellular infiltration and fatty infiltration ) (27); 3) persistent dyskinesia or tardive dyskinesia.

Persistent dyskinesia or tardive dyskinesia is a syndrome consisting of abnormal stereotyped involuntary movements of mouth, tongue, face, limbs and trunk, which occurs rather late in the course of drug treatment.

## Tardive Dyskinesia

*Diagnostic Criteria for Tardive Dyskinesia*

1.  The disorder is characterized by involuntary, stereotyped movements.
2.  These movements disappear during sleep.
3.  Involuntary efforts and activity of muscles in the affected areas can temporarily suppress the movements (28).

*High Risk Factors for Tardive Dyskinesia*

1.  The risk of tardive dyskinesia is higher in patients who have had long term neuroleptic therapy.
2.  Anticholinergic drugs may increase the likelihood of development of T.D.
3.  Tardive dyskinesia is more common in patients over 40.
4.  The prevalence of T.D. is greater among women than men.
5.  Patients who have brain damage tend to have a higher prevalence of tardive dyskinesia (28).

*Pathophysiology of Tardive Dyskinesia*

Neuroleptics reduce dopamine activity by blocking dopamine receptors. Prolonged administration of neuroleptics is presumed to produce a state of chemical denervation of dopamine receptors. To compensate for this, the postsynaptic dopamine neurons nigro-striatal system increases the number of dopamine receptors. When the neuroleptic induced blockade loses its effectiveness ( as a consequence of drug withdrawal or dose reduction or in some cases due to tolerance) a state of hyperactivity or hypersensitivity results. Another hypothesis suggests that there is a deficiency in the cholinergic transmission; experimentally the intravenous administration of physotigmine improves the abnormal movements of T.D. (29).

From the prognosis point of view there are two types of T.D.'s:

1.  The reversible that may be associated with only functional changes.
2.  The persistent dyskinesia or irreversible dyskinesia, occuring almost exclusively in elderly which appears to be associated with structural changes and may be related to

degenerative changes in dopaminergic, cholinergic or GABA–ergic systems, possible cell loss related both to age and neuroleptic treatment (28).

## Prevention of Tardive Dyskinesia

1. Use of neuroleptics only when they are indicated.
2. Prescribe them in the lowest effective doses.
3. Avoid unnecessary use of anticholinergic agents because lowering ACh increases the lack of equilibrium between DA and ACh.
4. Recent studies have found high positive correlation between T.D. and number of drug–free periods or in persons who have a history of interrupted drug treatment (30).

## Treatment

Due to the fact that the absolute etiological mechanism of T.D. is not fully understood, there is no agreement as to the most efficient way of handling the problem. It has been suggested that clonidine may produce improvement of T.D. (31). The possibility that T.D. is related to the deficiency of acetylcholine suggests that a possible treatment for T.D. is the administration of a precursor or acetylcholine such as Deanol® (32) and/or choline or lecithin (33).

## ADULT DOSAGE RANGE OF NEUROLEPTICS

|  | *Adult Dose* *(mg/day)* |
|---|---|
| **Phenothiazines** | |
|   Aliphatics | |
|     Chlorpromazine (Thorazine®) | 100–1600 mg |
| **Piperidines** | |
|     Thioridazine (Mellaril®) | 100–800 mg |
|     Mesoridazine (Serentil®) | 100–400 mg |
| **Piperazines** | |
|     Trifluoperazine (Stelazine®) | 2–30 mg |
|     Perphenazine (Trilafon®) | 2–64 mg |
|     Prochlorperazine (Compazine®) | 15–125 mg |
|     Fluphenazine (Prolixin–Permitil®) | 0.5–20 mg |
| **Thioxanthene Derivatives** | |
|     Chlorprothixene (Taractan®) | 40–600 mg |
|     Thiothixene (Navane®) | 6–60 mg |
| **Dibenzoxazepine Derivatives** | |
|     Loxapine Succinate (Loxitane®) | 20–250 mg |
| **Butyrophenones** | |
|     Haloperidol (Haldol®) | 3–50 mg |
| **Indole Derivatives** | |
|     Molindone HCL (Moban®) | 15–250 mg |
| **Rauwolfia Alkaloids** | |
|     Resperine (Sepasil®) | 1–5 mg |

<table>
<tr><td colspan="2" align="center">USUAL DOSAGES<br>FOR THE MOST FREQUENTLY PRESCRIBED NEUROLEPTICS<br>IN THE TREATMENT OF PSYCHOSIS</td></tr>
<tr><td></td><td align="right">Daily Dosage</td></tr>
<tr><td>Phenothiazines</td><td></td></tr>
<tr><td>  Aliphatics</td><td></td></tr>
<tr><td>    Chlorpromazine</td><td>100–1000 mg</td></tr>
<tr><td>Piperidines</td><td></td></tr>
<tr><td>    Thioridazine (Mellaril®)</td><td>100–800 mg</td></tr>
<tr><td>    Mesoridazine (Serentil®)</td><td>100–400 mg</td></tr>
<tr><td>Piperazines</td><td></td></tr>
<tr><td>    Trifluoperazine (Stelazine®)</td><td>2–30 mg</td></tr>
<tr><td>    Perphenazine (Trilafon®)</td><td>2–64 mg</td></tr>
<tr><td>    Prochlorperazine (Compazine®)</td><td>15–125 mg</td></tr>
<tr><td>    Fluphenazine (Prolixin–Permitil®)</td><td>0.5–20 mg</td></tr>
<tr><td>Thioxanthene Derivatives</td><td></td></tr>
<tr><td>    Thiothixene (Navane®)</td><td>6–60 mg</td></tr>
<tr><td>    Chlorprothixene (Taractan®)</td><td>10–600 mg</td></tr>
<tr><td>Dibenzoxazepine Derivatives</td><td></td></tr>
<tr><td>    Loxapine Succinate (Loxitane®)</td><td>20–250 mg</td></tr>
<tr><td>Butyrophenones</td><td></td></tr>
<tr><td>    Haloperidol (Haldol®)</td><td>3–50 mg</td></tr>
<tr><td>Indole Derivatives</td><td></td></tr>
<tr><td>    Molindone HCI (Moban®)</td><td>15–250 mg</td></tr>
<tr><td>Rauwolfia Alkaloids</td><td></td></tr>
<tr><td>    Reserpine (Serpasil®)</td><td>1–5 mg</td></tr>
</table>

Little or no rationale exists for combining two neuroleptics (10). Combination of a neuroleptic with a tricyclic antidepressant may create opposition in their crucial actions. Nonetheless, some studies have shown that patients seem to get the best of each drug in the combination (10).

## Overdosage and Toxicology

Signs and symptoms: hypotension, tachycardia, tachypnea, hypothermia, absent tendon reflexes, convulsions, coma and severe stomatitis. Usually the patient has to take high doses of neuroleptics (e.g., 6 gm of chlorpromazine or 3.75 gm of thioridazine) (34).

## Indications of Neuroleptics

1. Any type of schizophrenia (35, 36).
2. Schizophreniform disorders (37).
3. Paranoid disorders (37).
4. Brief reactive psychosis (37).
5. Manic episodes (37).
6. Major depression with psychotic features (4).
7. Agitation (even agitated depression, agitation due to brain syndromes or other types of medical illness) (38, 39).
8. Anorexia nervosa or brittle diabetes mellitus (due to the appetite stimulating properties) (4).
9. Acute intermittent porphyria (40).
10. Nausea and vomiting (2, 41).
11. The affective flattening which phenothiazine derivatives produce can be very useful in cases of intractable pain (41).
12. Chlorpromazine has been described as "the most effective agent ever introduced into therapy of intractable hiccup" (42).
13. Gilles de la Tourette's syndrome (41).

## Contraindications of the Neuroleptics

1. Allergy
2. CNS depression (coma, intoxication with CNS depressants).
3. Should be used with caution in narrow angle glaucoma due to anticholinergic action.
4. Should be used with caution in pregnancy during the first three months of pregnancy due to possible teratogenic effects.
5. Great care is necessary in administering the drugs to patients with severe cardiovascular disease, particularly marked hypotension or cardiac failure (9).
6. Bone marrow depression.

## ANTIDEPRESSANTS

The term antidepressant refers to drugs that moderate certain syndromes characterized by long lasting morbid sadness along with other manifestations. At the present time, we have four different kinds of antidepressants: the dibenzazepine derivatives or tricyclics, the MAO inhibitors, the tetracyclic antidepressants and the unclassified antidepressants.

Among the tricyclic antidepressants that are presently on the market in the USA are:

1. Imipramine hydrochloride (Tofranil®, Presamine®, Imavate®, Janimine®, Supramine®, Imipramine HCl®: doses 75–300 mg) and imipramine pamoate (Tofranil PM®: doses 75–300 mg qid).
2. Desipramine (Norpramin®, Petrograne®): daily doses 75–300 mg.
3. Amitriptyline HCl (Elavil®, Endep®): daily doses 75–300 mg.
4. Amozapine (Asendin®): daily doses 200–300 mg.
5. Trimipramine maleate (Surmontil®): doses 75–300 mg.
6. Nortriptyline (Aventyl®, Pamelor®): daily doses 20–300 mg.
7. Protriptyline (Vivactil®): daily doses 20–60 mg
8. Doxepine (Sinequan®, Adapin®): daily doses 75–150 mg

### Chemistry and Physiological Properties of Tricyclic Antidepressants

Tricyclic antidepressants bear strong structural resemblance to the tricyclic neuroleptics. The tricyclic compounds have two benzene rings joined through a central seven–member ring.

### Pharmacological Effects

1. They block the re–uptake of norepinephrine (mainly secondary amine metabolites, nortriptyline and desipramine) and serotonin (mainly the tertiary amines such as amitriptyline and imipramine) (43).
2. The have variable sedative effects, not too different from that of phenothiazines (more accentuated with amitriptyline and doxepin) (43).

3. They have potent central and peripheral anticholinergic action (43).
4. The tricyclic agents also weakly inhibit MAO (43).
5. They have antihistaminic effect (43).
6. It has been considered that either very low or very high levels of tricyclic antidepressants in the blood may be correlated with diminished effectivity (43). The quantitative analysis of these compounds have been done with the following results:

|  |  | Expected range |
|---|---|---|
| Amitriptyline | Therapeutic..... | 20-200 mg/ml |
|  | Toxic.......... | 100-200 mg/ml |
| Nortriptyline | Therapeutic..... | 30-120 mg/ml |
|  | Toxic.......... | 100-1200 mg/ml |
| Imipramine | Therapeutic..... | 20-160 mg/ml |
|  | Toxic.......... | 700-2000 mg/ml |
| Desipramine | Therapeutic..... | 15-65 mg/ml |
|  | Toxic.......... | 500-3000 mg/ml |

7. Research so far justifies that the dosage of tricyclic antidepressants does not reliably predict the effective concentration that will be attained in the blood.
8. There is a period of latency of 10-24 days before the therapeutic effect occurs.
9. Some drugs given concomitantly with tricyclic antidepressants can influence the therapeutic efficacy of the antidepressants.

## Substances that Raise Blood Levels of the Tricyclic Antidepressants

1. Methylphenidate (Ritalin®)
2. Disulfiram (Antabuse®)
3. Phenothiazines
4. Haloperidol
5. Morphine
6. Meperidine

## Substances that Lower the Blood Levels

1. Barbiturate hypnotics
2. Smoking
3. Alcohol

4. Insecticides
5. Fluthethimide (Doriden®)
6. Anticonvulsants
7. Meprobramate

## Possible Mechanism of Action of Antidepressants

As stated before, 1) imipramine and amitriptyline have been shown to block uptake of serotonin into the presynaptic terminal; 2) desipramine and nortriptyline have a more potent inhibition in the reuptake of norepinephrine; 3) also, anticholinergic properties may play a role in improving the manifestations of depression; 4) the antihistaminic activity of these drugs may contribute to the improvement of certain manifestations of depression; 5) in regard to NE, they decrease the postsynaptic B–adrenergic receptor sensitivity; 6) cortisol production is excessive in about 50% of patients with depression, and the antidepressants appear to reduce it in multiple cases (43, 45).

## Side Effects

Tricyclic antidepressants and tricyclic neuroleptics have many side effects in common. Hypersensitivity reactions such as jaundice and skin reactions are the same.

<br>

| AUTONOMIC SIDE EFFECTS | |
| --- | --- |
| *More Frequently* | *Less Frequently* |
| Dry mouth | Hypersalivation |
| Tachycardia | Bradycardia |
| Constipation | Diarrhea |
| Perspiration | Anhydrosis |
| Postural hypotension | Hypertension |
| Hyperthermia | Hypothermia |
| Pollakiuria | Urinary Retention |
| Mydriasis | Miosis |

### Quindine–like Effects of the Tricyclics

Palpitations, tachycardia, and arrhythmias are not unusual. EKG changes include prolongation of the QT interval and flattening of the T wave. The myocardium is often directly depressed.

### Intestinal Symptoms

These compounds can produce constipation and diarrhea, anorexia and increased appetite, nausea and vomiting. Moreover, the tricyclics have been implicated in the worsening of hiatus hernias.

### Endocrinological Effects

Galactorrhea, weight gain, decreased blood sugar and decreased glycosuria in diabetic patients.

### Hematopoietic Effects

Leukopenia, eosinophilia, agranulocytosis, aplastic anemia (may occur).

### Neurological Side Effects

Tremor (after large doses) paresthesias, disturbance in coordination and muscular weakness, convulsions (usually with high doses).

### Psychiatric Effects

Insomnia, hypersomnia, hypomanic and manic states, paranoid and auditory hallucinatory pictures, visual hallucination, hypnogogic hallucinations, and the most striking psychiatric complication is delirium.

## Withdrawal Reactions

Restlessness, anxiety, akathisia.

## Overdosage

Infants and older persons are more sensitive to these drugs. 575 mg of TAD may be fatal in a two-year-old child and 1000 mg can be fatal for an old person. Fatalities have been reported from 1250 mg to 2500 mg in adults.

## Manifestations of Intoxication

Tremors, anxiety, myclonic movements, hypotension, cardiac complications, anuria, mydriasis, reflex changes, convulsions, cyanois and coma (9).

## Indications for the Use of Tricyclic Antidepressants

1. Any type of depression, but mainly major depressions (43).
2. Anxiety, mainly panic disorders (46)
3. Narcolepsy (47)
4. Enuresis nocturna (48)
5. Attention deficit disorder or hyperkinetic syndrome or minimal brain dysfunction (49)
6. Encorpresis (50)
7. Some cases of school phobias (51)
8. Obsessive compulsive phobic disorders (46)
9. May be helpful in some pain syndromes that might represent "depressive equivalents" (52).
10. Migraine (53)

## Contraindication of the Tricyclic Antidepressants

1. Allergy
2. CNS depression
3. Should be used with caution in narrow angle glaucoma and pregnancy.
4. Close supervision of patients with hyperthyroidism or those receiving thyroid medication.
5. Drugs are not recommended during acute recovery phase following myocardial infarction.

6. Severe convulsion and hyperpiretic crises and death have been reported with combination of tricyclic antidepressants and MAO inhitibors.
7. Acute relapses have been reported in schizophrenic patients.

## Combination of Tricyclic Antidepressants and Other Drugs

It has been postulated that the combination of lithium carbonate and tricyclic antidepressants may be effective in cases of bipolar disorders when the patient develops depression; other people have denied this effectivity (54).

The use of small amounts of thyroid hormone combined with imipramine in patients unresponsive to imipramine alone has been recommended (55).

Methylphenidate increases tricyclic plasma level (56).

Tricyclic antidepressants increase anticholinergic activity of anticholinergic drugs (57).

## MAO INHIBITORS

The MAO inhibitors are a group of agents with the common property of inhibiting a class of enzymes designated as the mono amine oxidase. Among them we find the following:

Phenelzine sulfate (Nardil®): daily doses 45–75 mg

Isocarboxazid (Marplan®): daily doses 10–30 mg

Tranylcypromine sulfate (Parnate®): daily doses 20–30 mg

The MAO inhibitors not only inhibit the metabolism of catecholamines in the brain but also inhibit the metabolism of other amines in other parts of the body, and also inhibit the metabolism of numerous drugs. The inhibition of the metabolosm of tyramine which increases the release or norepinephrine may cause hypertension. Patient must follow strict diets avoiding foods that contain tyramine, among them are the following: beer, wine (especially chianti), other alcoholic beverages in large amounts, some cheeses, yeast supplements, smoked or pickled fish (herring), ripe avocado, beef or chicken liver, large amounts of sour cream, summer dry sausage, soy sauce, fava or broad beans pods, large amounts of yogurt.

## Side Effects

The most common side effects related to the MAO inhibitors are: orthostatic hypotension, dizziness, jitteriness, insomnia, hypertensive crises as mentioned above, induction of mania and heptacellular jaundice (rare).

## Contraindications

Phenochromocytoma, significant liver disease, upcoming general anesthesia and cerebrovascular disease.

## Indications

These drugs are not first choice drug treatment for any indications. Sometimes they are useful for disorders refractory to tricyclics, especially: atypical depression, panic disorder, agoraphobia, obsessive compulsive disorders and narcolepsy (58).

# TETRACYCLIC ANTIDEPRESSANTS

These are compounds with a basic structure of four coupled rings.

Maprotiline (Ludiomil®):  150–300 mg daily oral dose

Pharmaceutically, this drug is important in that it is a potent inhibitor of the re-uptake of NE and does not affect the serotonin system. It seems to have an early onset of antidepressive action. The side effects are similar to the tricyclic antidepressants (59).

# UNCLASSIFIED ANTIDEPRESSANTS

The only one available in the USA is trazodone (Desyrel®). It has been stated that trazodone has a considerable anxiolitic action, in fact equal to diazepam and chlordiazepoxide. Trazodone resembles the benzodiazepines more than the antidepressants on the basis of the EEG (60). Excellent tolerance has also been reported. The significant biochemical actions of trazodone are selective inhibition of 5-hydroxitryptamine (5HT) uptake and interaction with 5HT binding sites. Average dose: 150–600 mg.

## Side Effects

In regard to autonomic nervous system, cardiovascular, genitourinary, allergies, etc., trazodone shows less tendency to cause them. The only consistently noted side effects are drowsiness and slight sedation a few hours after intake (61).

# MINOR TRANQUILIZERS

Minor tranquilizers are a group of different drugs that include the benzodiazepines, propanediols, antihistamines and some barbiturates and beta blockers. They are used for their antianxiety properties. They are also called anxiolitics, day time sedatives and calmatives. Except for the antihistamine group and beta blockers, they show some common properties.

1. They are anxiolitics (62).
2. They produce some kind of immediate lift (4).
3. They cause diminished arousal response to different stimuli
4. They have anticonvulsant properties (62).
5. The produce slow–waves and low voltage fast (beta) activity in the EEG (63).
6. They are hypnotics (62).
7. Like CNS depressants, they cause the person who takes them to become tolerant of their hypnotic and tranquilizing effects simultaneously (4).
8. Abrupt withdrawal of these drugs after protracted use produces similar symptoms as are seen after withdrawal from other CNS depressants (4).
9. They exhibit cross tolerance and cross dependence with other CNS depressants.
10. They are often used in excess by individuals who have in the past abused other CNS depressants (4).
11. They have muscle relaxant properties (62).

The most commonly prescribed anxiolytic drugs are presented in the table below.

## COMMONLY PRESCRIBED ANXIOLYTIC DRUGS

| Drug | Dispositional Half-Life | Active Metabolites | Dosage Per Day |
|---|---|---|---|
| **BENZODIAZEPINES** | | | |
| Short-acting | | | |
| Triazolam | 1.7–2.3 hrs | hydroxytriazolam & 4hydroxytriazolam | 0.25–0.5 mg |
| Oxazepam | 5–15 hrs. | None | 15–120 mg |
| Lorazepam | 10–20 hrs. | None | 2–4 mg |
| Temazepam | 10 hrs. | None | 15–30 mg |
| Halazepam | 14 hrs. | N–demethyldiazepam | 40–160 mg |
| Alprazolam | 12–15 hrs. | hydroxyalprezolam | 0.25–4 mg |
| Moderately long-acting | | | |
| Diazepam | 26–53 hrs. | N–desmethyldiazepam | 40–160 mg |
| Chlordiazepoxide | 8–28 hrs. | Several | 10–200 mg |
| Long-acting | | | |
| Clorazepate | 30–200 hrs. | N–desmethyldiazepam | 20–60 mg |
| Prazepam | | | |
| Very long-acting | | | |
| Flurazepam | 96+ hrs. | N–desalkylflurazepam | 15–30 mg |
| **PROPANEDIOLS** | | | |
| Meprobamate (Miltown®, Equanil®, etc.) | | | 200–2000 mg |
| Tyabamate (Tybatran®) | | | 250–2800 mg |
| **ANTIHISTAMINES** | | | |
| Hydroxyzine (Vistaril® or Atarax®) | | | 30–400 mg |
| Diphenydramine (Benadryl®) | | | 50–300 mg |
| **ADRENERGIC ANTAGONISTS** | | | |
| Propanolol (Inderal®) (not yet approved by FDA as an anxiolytic) | | | 10–240 mg |

## Benzodiazepines

Benzodiazepines seem to be superior to the rest of the anxiolytics for the treatment of chronic anxiety (64, 65). They produce less severe withdrawal symptoms than the others and convulsions occur only in the rarest of instances (4). They cause little respiratory depression, even when used in massive doses, so successful suicide is rare with benzodiazepines alone (4). Unlike barbiturates and propanediol derivatives, benzodiazepines do not markedly stimulate hepatic microsomal metabolic enzymes so they are less likely to lose effectiveness when taken for a long period of time.

Some of the benzodiazepines have a long duration action (chlordiazepoxide: 8–24 hours; diazepam: 20–50 hours). Elimination half-life hours up to 200 hours (prazepam). Benzodiazepines have low risk of producing physical tolerance, but they produce habituation (66). In high intravenous doses, they produce anterograde amnesia (66).

## Biochemical Action Mechanism

These compounds appear to reduce the turnover of noradrenaline (NA) as well as that of dopamine (DA) and serotonin (SHT), and they reduce the stress-induced increase in central NA turnover. Benzodiazepines are believed to potentiate effects of GABA-energic neurons. This effect is believed to be involved in at least three benzodiazepine activities:

1. Muscle relaxation
2. Anticonvulsant activity
3. Ataxia, which can be a side effect of benzodiazepines given in large doses.

There are indications that benzodiazepines interact with post-synaptic glycine receptors (65).

## Propanediols

Propanediols have been used less frequently lately because: 1) they have a narrow margin between therapeutic and lethal doses; 2) frequently meprobamate is associated with physical dependence; 3) tolerance may develop with severe withdrawal manifestations; and 4) they are less effective than benzodiazepines (44).

## Antihistamine Minor Tranquilizers

These may be of value in treatment of anxiety and related skin conditions. They can be used in individuals who are prone to become drug addicts. However, their therapeutic response is unpredictable and they at times precipitate paradoxical excitement. Furthermore, tolerance may develop to their pharmacological effects (44).

Postulated way and site of action: There are many hypotheses, but these have not yet been proven.

Beta blockers (propanediol) in a daily dose of 40 to 100 mg is particularly effective when anxiety is manifested mostly in somatic symptoms (67).

## Clinical Indications (Mainly of the Benzodiazepines)

1. Acute and chronic anxiety (37)
2. Phobias (37)
3. Adjustment disorder with anxious mood (37)
4. Management of alcohol withdrawal (68)
5. Neurological disorders (status epilepticus doses up to 100 mg of diazepam in 50 cc of saline; athetoid cerebral palsy; suppress sustained alkeclonus in quadriparetics (69)
6. Tetanus (70)
7. Pain due to muscle strain in disc disease (69)
8. As preanesthetic medication (to relieve anxiety) (71)
9. In cardioversion (to relieve anxiety and tension) (72)
10. As hypnotics (short acting benzodiazepines may be recommended) (64).

## Side Effects of Minor Tranquilizers

Drowsiness, vertigo, excessive appetite, paradoxical nausea and vomiting, muscular weakness, impaired judgment, poor coordination, cerebellar type of ataxia, and hypotension are the more common side effects of these drugs. They also potentiate action of narcotics (71).

## Contraindications

Allergy to the drugs, coma, questionable contraindication in narrow angle glaucoma. They are also contraindicated in acute alcoholic intoxication with depression of vital signs. They should be used with caution in pregnancy. They are also contraindicated in myasthenia gravis and ataxia.

## STIMULANTS

Stimulants are compounds with central stimulating effects which become manifested mostly in increased motor activity and euphoria. In general, they activate the sympathetic nervous system and they tend to produce: mydriasis, hypertension, relaxation of intestinal muscles, decrease coagulation, increase blood sugar level, contract urinary bladder sphincter, decrease the blood coagulation time, increase tone and contractibility of skeletal muscle, produce wakefulness, decrease feeling of fatigue, decrease appetite, some increase in analgesic activity and stimulation in the respiratory center. They also may produce changes in the EEG characterized by low voltage and fast activity (73).

### Classification

1. Amphetamine derivatives, i.e., compounds with phenylethylamine ring. The principal amphetamine derivatives at the present time are:
   a. Amphetamine (Benzedrine®) 5–20 mg average daily oral dose
   b. Dextroamphetamine (Dexedrine®) 5–20 mg average daily oral dose
   c. Methamphetamine (Desoxin®, Methedrine®) 3–12 mg average daily dose
2. Compounds with a piperidine ring
   a. Methylphenidate (Ritalin®) 20–30 mg average daily dose
   b. Pipadrol (Meratran®) 3–7.5 mg average daily dose
3. Oxazolidine compounds: Pemolin (Cylert®) 18.5–112.5 mg average daily dose
4. Oxazine group: Phenmetrazine (Preludin®) 25–75 average daily dose
5. Deanol (Deaner®) 250–500 mg average daily dose.

The latter does not depress the appetite, blood pressure, pulse rate and does not cause jitteriness.

**Biochemical Effects (Except for Deanol)**

1. Release of catecholamines from presynaptic area
2. Block reuptake of catecholamines
3. Possibility of mimicking the action of catecholamines
4. They have some MAO inhibitor action (41).

**Toxicity**

1. Acute toxicity: greater magnitude of their pharmacological effects (usually with excessive doses) along with manifestations of delirium.
2. Chronic toxicity: similar manifestations as acute paranoid schizophrenia (73).

**Indications of the Stimulants**

The use of stimulants is justifiable in the following conditions:

1. Narcolepsy
2. Minimal brain dysfunction
3. Control of hypnotic effects of certain antiepileptic agents
4. As an adjunct to narco-analytic treatment
5. Nocturnal enuresis, but in view of the rapidly developing tolerance, the efficacy of this treatment is very doubtful.

**Dangers and Side Effects**

1. Addiction (fashionable way of becoming high). Tolerance to central stimulating effects occur and patients develop depression after discontinuing the stimulants if they had been taken for a long period of time.
2. Sleep disturbance
3. Acute anxiety
4. Anorexia
5. Except in case of massive doses, stimulants exert no influence on convulsive threshold (41, 73).

## Contraindications of the Stimulants (Except for Deanol)

Cardiovascular (advanced arteriosclerosis) hypertension, hyperthyroidism, hypersensitivity to the drugs, agitated states, drug dependence, pregnancy. Due to the fact that these drugs are potentially addicting, the use in obesity is not justified.

## LITHIUM

John Cade (1) in 1949 proved the effectiveness of lithium as an antimanic drug. At the present time, lithium carbonate and lithium citrate are the only salt of lithium that have been approved in the USA for the treatment of the manic phase of bipolar disorders.

It is not known why lithium is highly specific in alleviating the manic manifestations of bipolar depressive disorder, but among its biological effect we found: 1) It competes with Na+ Mg++ and Ca++, affecting electrolyte balance and transport. It may also interact with ammonium groups, including those of the biogenic amines. 2) May alter hormones that regulate electrolyte balance such as aldosterone, elevating it. 3) Indications have been found that lithium reduces the amount of NE at the central post-synaptic receptors by inhibiting its release and increasing its reuptake. 4) At the beginning, lithium has been shown to increase L-tryptophan uptake with subsequent increase in 5–HT synthesis. However, after chronic treatment, 5–HT synthesis is believed to be stabilized. 5) It also increases intracellular turnover of catecholamines. 6) It appears to inhibit activity of adenylate cyclase. 7) Lithium also may block the development of supersensitive neuronal receptors. 8) Lithium is known to modify the high affinity binding of agonists and antagonists of opiate receptors and also, it has been reported that lithium increases striatal encephalin content (74).

## Doses

Usual dose in acute mania is from 1200 to 2400 mg daily in divided doses. In the market, we find 300 mg tablets or capsule, slow releasing tablets and syrup citrate.

Blood lithium level should never be above 2 mEq/liter. Once therapeutic levels have been reached, dosage should be determined on the third, seventh and fourteenth day to establish levels between 0.7 and 1.2 mEq/liter. Later on, lithium levels should be checked every month or every three months.

## Side Effects

### CNS Effects

1. Slowing of EEG
2. Chronic low dosage of Li exacerbated temporal lobe epilepsy or may promoke grand mal seizures.
3. Mild neurological effects more common at the start of the treatment include: fatigue, lethargy, muscle weakness and tremor.
4. Moderate neurological effects, usually dose related, include: muscular hyperirritability, extrapyramidal manifestations, ataxia, coarsening of tremor, dysarthria, incoordination, difficulty concentrating, disorientation, confusion, altered level of consciousness and visual disturbances.
5. Severe neurological manifestations: any of the signs or symptoms mentioned before may progress in severity to coma, seizures, delirium, brain damage and even death (75).
6. Lithium reduced REM sleep.
7. Lithium may adversely effect the symptoms of myasthenia gravis.

### Renal Effects

Lithium produces two distinct categories of renal effects:
1. The most frequent and most benign effect is a vasopressin-resistant diabetes insipidus-like syndrome.
2. More alarming with chronic lithium intake, there could be renal damage via direct and presumably irreversible nephrotoxic effect.

### Hemotologic Effects

1. Most patients develop a relative leukocytosis.
2. It does not appear to interfere with blood coagulation.

3. Lithium therapy should not be a contraindication for donating blood (75).

*Cardiovascular Effects*

1. Benign, reversible electrocardiographic T waves (resembling hypokalemia).
2. Sometimes premature ventricular contractions and sinus node arrhythmias.
3. There does not appear to be a higher than expected incidence of cardiovasuclar malformations in lithium babies with high occurrence of Ebstein's anomaly of the tricuspid valve.
4. In the presence of lithium intoxication, arrhythmias, hypotension and vascular collapse are more commonly seen.
5. There has been epidemiological speculation that a high lithium content in drinking water may be related to the decreased incidence of arteriosclerotic heart disease (75).

*Metabolic and Endocrinologic Effects*

1. Weight gain (from 10% to 33% of the cases).
2. Lithium has complex effects on carbohydrate metabolism. Both increased and decreased glucose tolerance have been shown in men; but its use in diabetics is not contraindicated.
3. a) Lithium produces a generally benign diminution in the concentration of circulating thyroid hormones. b) In about 3.6% of patients treated for more than six months, enlargement of the thyroid gland has been found, with or without hypothyroidism or hypothyroidism with or without enlargement of the thyroid gland. c) Lithium inhibits TSH induced thyroid response and it may produce exaggerated TSH response to TRH stimulation. d) The most consistent effect of lithium at therapeutic levels is to inhibit iodine release including $T_3$ and $T_4$ from the thyroid gland. e) Sometimes exophthalmus may appear.

With the exception of its effects on the thyroid, lithium has not been shown to have a consistent effect on other hormones.

*Dermatological Effects*

In general, lithium therapy is not associated with notable dermatological manifestations, however, there have been reports of maculopapular rashes, alopecia, pruritic dermatitis, ulceration and acne-like dermatological manifestations (75, 76, 77).

*Teratogenic Effects*

Actual percentage of malformation in the International Register of Lithium Babies (babies whose mothers took lithium during their pregnancy) is 11%; more than three-fourths of them had cardiac malformations. Lithium clearance increases during pregnancy by 50% to 100%. The clearance returns to normal at the time of delivery, if no reduction of lithium dose is made at the time of delivery, toxicity may ensue (75, 76, 77).

*Gastrointestinal Effects*

Initiation of lithium treatment is frequently accompanied by abdominal discomfort such as: gastric irritation, epigastric bloating or pressure, abdominal pain, nausea, emesis, anorexia and diarrhea. Gradual and deliberate dosage schedule may diminish or help these manifestations (75, 76, 77).

## Lithium Poisoning

Since the art of lithium pharmacotherapy has become refined, intoxication is far less common. Lithium intoxication may be related to accidental or deliberate overdose, impaired renal function, diuretic therapy, salt restriction, dehydration, inter-current illness or childbirth. Permanent neurological damage or death may be the result.

## Treatment of Lithium Intoxication

At the present time in the USA, the only way to administer lithium for therapeutic purpose is by mouth. The kidney is the only important route of lithium excretion. Lithium is eliminated from the body within ten to twelve days. The severity of lithium poisoning correlates both with the magnitude of serum lithium concentration and with the length of time a person is exposed to those concentrations.

A negative Na balance causes a decrease in lithium clearance since lithium is absorbed with Na in the proximal tubule.

## General Measures to Treat Lithium Intoxication

1. Physical and psychiatric monitoring (intensive care).
2. Gastric emptying.
3. Increasing renal clearance (if reduced clearance is due to a negative Na balance, the administration of Na chloride should result in improvement).
4. Dialysis: both peritoneal dialysis and hemodialysis are quite effective in removing lithium from the body. They should be used as soon as possible if serum lithium is higher than 4 mEq/liter even if clinical state is stable or if serum lithium level is between 2 and 4 mEq/liter and clinical condition is poor. If dialysis is not available, the use of osmotic diuretics, aminophylline, acetazolamid and Na bicarbonate that increase excretion of lithium by 30–60% may be of value.
5. Correction of fluid and electrolyte imbalance (75).

## Indications for Lithium Therapy

1. Bipolar disorders
2. Schizaffective Disorder, manic type (75) (possibly in combination with neuroleptics)
3. Intermittent explosive disorders (76)
4. Cyclothymic disorders (37)

## Contraindications for Lithium Therapy

Lithium should not be given to patients with significant renal or cardiovascular disease, severe debilitation or dehydration or sodium depletion and to patients receiving diuretics. The risk of lithium toxicity is very high in such patients. If the psychiatric condition is life threatening and the patients have failed to respond to other measures, lithium should be given with extreme caution and hospitalization. But none of these conditions represent fatal contraindications.

## REFERENCES

1. Cade JIJ: Lithium salts in the treatment of psychotic excitement. Med J Aust, 2:349–352, 1949.

2. Delay J, Deniker P: Trente–huit case de psychoses traitees par la cure prolongee et continuee de 4560 RF, Le Congres des al et Neurol et Langue Fr in Compte Rendue du Congres. Paris: Masson et cie, 1952.

3. Baldessarini RJ: Chemotherapy in Psychiatry. Cambridge, MA: Harvard University Press, 1977.

4. Detre TP, Jarecki HG: Modern Psychiatric Treatment. Philadelphia: J.B. Lippincott Co., 1971.

5. Klerman GL, et al.: Sedation and tranquilization: comparison of effects of number of psychopharmacological agents upon normal human objects. Arch Gen Psychia, 3:4–13, 1960.

6. Szatmari A: Clinical and electroencephelogram investigation on largactil in psychoses (preliminary study). Amer J Psychia, 112:788–794, 1956.

7. Battegay R: Drug dependence as criterion for differentiation of psychotropic drugs. Compr Psychia, 7:501–509, 1966.

8. Logothetis J: Spontaneous epileptic seizures and electroencephalographic changes in the course of phenothiazine therapy. Neurology, 17:869, 1967.

9. Kalinowsky LB, Hippius H, Klein HE: Biological Treatments in Psychiatry. New York: Grune & Stratton, 1982.

10. Hollister LE: Clinical Pharmacology of Psychotherapeutic Drugs. New York: Churchill Livingston, 1978.

11. Miller RJ, Horn AS, Iversen LL: The action of neuroleptic drugs on dopamine stimulated adenosine cyclic 3'5' monophosphate production in neostriatum and limbic forebrain. Mod Pharmacol, 10:759–766, 1974.

12. Andrew NE, Stock C: Effect of clozapine on the turnover of dopamine in the corpus striatum and the limbic system. J Pharm Pharmacol, 344–348, 1973.

13. Khazan N, Primo C, Danon A, Sulman FG, Winnik HZ: The mammotropic effects of tranquilizing drugs. Archives Internationales de Pharmacodynamics et de Therapie, 141:291, 1962.

14. Carlsson A: Mechanism of action of neuroleptic drugs. In Lipton MA, DiMascio A, Killam KF (eds), Psychopharmacology: A Generation of Progress. New York: Raven Press, 1978, pp. 1057–1070.

15. Ayd FJ Jr.: Survey of drug-induced extrapyramidal reactions. JAMA, 175:1054–1060, 1961.

16. Schaaf M, Payne CA: Dystonic reactions to prochlorperazine in hypoparathyroidism. New Eng J Med, 275:991–995, 1966.

17. Freedman DX, DeJong J: Factors that determine drug-induced akathisia. Dis Nerv Syst, 22(Suppl.):69–76, 1971.

18. Klawans HL: Disorders of the extrapyramidal system. In Cohen MM (ed), Biochemistry of Neural Disease. New York: Harper & Row, 1975.

19. Rann WE, Lake CR: Amantadine versus trihexyphenidyl in the treatment of neuroleptic-induced parkinsonism. Am J Psychiatry, 133:940-943, 1976.

20. DiMascio A, Bernardo DL, Greenblatt, DJ, Mender JE: A controlled trial of amantadine in drug-induced extrapyramidal disorders. Arch Gen Psychia, 33:599, 1976.

21. Jacobson G. Baldessarini RJ, Manschreck T: Tardive and withdrawal dyskinesia associated with Haloperidol. Am J Psychia, 131:910-913, 1974.

22. Cohen IM: Complications of chlorpromazine therapy. Am J Psychia, 113:115, 1956.

23. Blair D, Brady DM: Recent advances in the treatment of schizophrenia: group training and tranquilizers. J Ment Sc, 104:625, 1958.

24. Gerle B: Clinical observations of the side effects of Haloperidol. Acta Psychia Scand, 40:65, 1964.

25. Dencker SJ, Enoksson P, Person PS: Pigment deposits in various organs during phenothiazine treatment, Acta Psychia Scand, 43:21-31, 1966.

26. Hagopian V, Stratton DB, Busiek RD: Five cases of pigmentary retinopathy associated with thioridazine administration. Amer J Psychia, 123: 97-100, 1966.

27. Hollister LE, Hall RA: Phenothiazine derivatives and morphological changes in the liver. Amer H Psychia, 123:211-212, 1966.

28. Fann W, Smith RC, David J, Domino E: Tardive Dyskinesia Research & Treatment. New York: S.O. Medical & Scientific Books, 1980.

29. Weis KJ, Ciraule DA, Shader RI: Physostigmine test in the rabbit syndrome and tardive dyskinesia. Amer J Psychia, 137:627-628, 1980.

30. Annath J. Tardive Dyskinesia: myths and realities. Psychosomatic, 21: 389-396, 1980.

31. Freedman R, Bell J, Kirch D: Clonidine therapy for co-existing psychosis and tardive dyskinesia. Am J Psychia, 137:629-630, 1980.

32. Penovich P, Morgan JP, Kerzner B, et al.: Double blind evaluation of deanol in tardive dyskinesia. JAMA, 239:1997-1998, 1978.

33. Wurtman RJ: Nutritional and precursor control of brain acetylcholine synthesis. Psychopharmacol Bull, 14:53-55, 1978.

34. Davis JM, Bartlett E, Termini BA: Overdosage of psychotropic drugs: a review. Part I: Major & minor tranquilizers. Part II: Antidepressants and other psychotropic agents. Dis Nerv Sys, 29:157 & 246, 1968.

35. Prien RF, Cole JO: High dose chlorpromazine therapy in chronic schizophrenia. Arch Gen Psychia, 18:482-495, 1968.

36. National Institute of Mental Health (Collaborative Study Group): Phenothiazine treatment in acute schizophrenia: effectiveness. Arch Gen Psych, 10:246-261, 1963.

37. Kaplan HI, Freedman AM, Sadock BJ (eds): Comprehensive Textbook of Psychiatry, Vol. II. Baltimore/London: Williams Wilkins, 1980.

38. Raskin A, et al.: Differential response to chlorpromazine, imipramine and placebo: a study of subgroups of hospitalized depressed patients. Arch Gen Psychiat, 23:164-173, 1970.

39. Blachly PH, Starr A: Treatment of delirium with phenothiazine drugs following open heart surgery. Dis Nerv Sys, 27(Suppl.):107-110, 1966.

40. Kolb LC, Brodie H, Keith H (eds): Modern Clinical Psychiatry. Philadelphia: W.B. Saunders Co., 1982.

41. Van Praag HM (ed): Psychotropic Drugs: A Guide for the Practitioner. New York: Brunner/Mazel, 1978.

42. Beckman H: Pharmacology. Philadelphia/London, W.B. Saunders, 1961.

43. Mendels J. Amsterdam JD (eds): The Psychobiology of Affective Disorders. Munchen: S. Krager Basel, 1980.

44. Barchase JD (ed): Psychopharmacology: From Theory to Practice. New York: Oxford University Press, 1977.

45. Enna SJ, Malick JB, Richelson E (eds): Antidepressants: Neurochemical, Behavioral & Clinical Perspectives. New York: Raven Press, 1981.

46. Sheehan DV: Current views on the treatment of pain & phobic disorders. Drug Therapy, October:74-93, 1982.

47. Akimoto H, Honda Y, Takahashi Y: Pharmacotherapy of narcolepsy. Dis Nerv Sys, 21:704, 1960.

48. McLean REG: Imipramine hydrochloride (Tofranil) and enuresis. Am J Psychia, 117:551, 1960.

49. Brown D, Winsberg BG, Bialer I, Press M: Imipramine therapy and seizures: three children treated for hyperactive behavior disorder. Am J Psychia, 130:210-212, 1973.

50. Schunzelar K: Treatment of enuresis and encopresis with Trofranil in chronic psychiatric female inpatients. Acta Neurol Psychia Belg, 63:333, 1963.

51. Gittelmann-Klein R, Klein DF: School phobia: diagnostic considerations in the light of imipramine effects. J Nerv Ment Dis, 156:199-215, 1973.

52. Taub A: Psychotropic drugs relieve post herpetic neuralgia. J Neurosurg, 39:335-339, 1973.

53. Gomersall JD, Stuart A: Amitriptyline in migraine prophylaxis: changes in pattern of attacks during a controlled clinical trial. J Neurolsurg & Psychia, 36:684-690, 1973.

54. Quitkin FM, Kane J, Rifkin A, Ramos-Lorenzi JR, Nayak DV: Prophylactic lithium carbonate with or without imipramine for bipolar 1 patients: double-blind study. Arch Gen Psychia, 38:902-907, August, 1981.

55. Goodwin FK, Prange AJ, Post RM, Giovani M. Potentiation of antidepressant effects by triiodothyronine in tricyclic nonresponders. Am J Psychia, 139:34-38, January, 1982.

56. Clark WG, Giudice J (eds): Principles of Psychopharmacology (second edition). New York/San Francisco/London: Academic Press, 1978.

57. Avery GS (ed): Drug Treatment: Principles & Practice of Clinical Pharmacology & Therapeutics (2nd Edition). Sidney/NewYork, Adis Press, 1980.

58. Lipton MA, DiMascio A, Killman KF (eds): Pharmacology: A Generation of Progress. New York: Raven Press, 1978.

59. Delini-Stula A: The pharmacology of ludiomil. In Kielholz (ed), Depressive Illness, Diagnosis, Assessment, Treatment. Bern Hans, Huber, 1972, pp. 113-124.

60. Cassano GB, Ghiozzi M, Fornaro P: Clinical experience with Trazodone. In Morozov G, Saarma J. Silvestrini B (eds), Depression and the Role of Trazodone in Antidepressant Therapy. Rome: Edizioni Luigi Pozzi SPA, 1978.

61. Feighner JP: Clinical efficacy of the newer antidepressants. J Clin Psychophar (Suppl.)I(6):235-265, 1981.

62. Skolnick P, Mendelson B, Paul SM: Benzodiazepines receptors in the CNS. Wheatley D (ed), Psychopharmacology of Sleep. New York: Raven Press, 1981.

63. Brazier MAB: Effect of drugs on the electroencephelogram of man. Clin Pharmacol Ther, 5:102-116, 1964.

64. Wheatley D: Chlordiazepoxide in the treatment of the domiciliary case of anxiety neurosis. Excerpta Med Internat Congr Series No. 150 (Proceedings of the IV World Congress of Psychiatry, Madrid, 1966) pp. 2034-2037.

65. Costa E, Greengard P (eds): Mechanism of Action of Benzodiazepines. New York: Raven Press, 1975.

66. Priest RD, Vianna Filho U, Amrei R, Skreta M (eds): Benzodiazepines Today and Tomorrow. Baltimore: University Park Press, 1980.

67. Kelly D: Clinical review of beta blockers in psychiatry. In Kielholz P (ed), A Therapeutic Approach to the Psyche via the B Adrenergic System. Baltimore: University Park Press, 1978.

68. Sereny G, Kalant H: Comparative clinical evaluation of chlordiazepoxide and promazine in the treatment of alcohol withdrawal syndrome. Brit Med J, 1:92-97, 1965.

69. Browne TR, Feldman RG: Clinical experiences of benzodiazepines in neurological disorders. In Priest RG (ed), Benzodiazepines Today and Tomorrow. Baltimore: University Park Press, 1980.

70. Haefely WE: Biological basis of the therapeutic effect of benzodiazepines. In Priest RG (ed), Benzodiazepines Today and Tomorrow. Baltimore: University Park Press, 1980.

71. Greenblatt DJ, Shader RI (eds): Benzodiazepines in Clinical Practice. New York: Raven Press, 1974.

72. Kelly D: Clinical experiences with benzodiazepines in psychosomatic disorders. In Priest RG (ed): Benzodiazepines Today and Tomorrow. Baltimore: University Park Press, 1980.

73. Kornetsky C (ed): Pharmacology: Drugs Affecting Behavior. New York: John Wiley & Sons, 1976.

74. Bunney WB, Pert A, Rosemblatt J, Pert CB, Gallaper D: Mode of action of lithium: some biological considerations. Arch Gen Psychia, 36:898-901, July 1979.

75. Jefferson JW, Creist JH (eds): The Primer of Lithium Therapy. Baltimore: Williams & Wilkins Co., 1977.

76. Sheard MH, Marini JL, Bridges CI, et al.: The effect of lithium on impulsive aggressive behavior in man. Am J Psychia, 133:1409-1413, 1976.

77. Gershon S, Shopsin B: Lithium: Its Role in Psychiatric Research & Treatment. New York: Plenum Publishing Copr., 1973.

# Chapter 12

## ELECTROCONVULSIVE THERAPY

## OCTAVIO C. PINELL, M.D.

Electroconvulsive therapy (ECT) is an empirically derived treatment developed in the 1930s and used in several psychiatric conditions, e.g., depression and schizophrenia. Since its introduction, this procedure has been the object of exaggerated praise as well as extreme vilification (1). In fact, ECT is neither a panacea nor a form of medieval torture. Its judicious administration is an important and sometimes life-saving psychiatric treatment that may offer substantial symptomatic relief, particularly for the severely ill.

Electricity is not necessary to produce therapeutic convulsions. In 1785, Oliver induced therapeutic convulsions with camphor; in 1933, Von Meduna revived the technique, but because of many drawbacks (sometimes it did not produce convulsions, sometimes it produced several convulsions), Von Meduna was led to use pentylenetetrazol (Metrazol®) I.V. in 1957, Krantz introduced hexafluorodiethyl ether, a convulsant drug called Indoklon® which was used mainly by inhalation. This treatment appears equally as effective as Metrazol® or ECT (2).

Cerletty and Bini (3) in 1938 introduced the use of electrically induced convulsions which has been called electroconvulsive therapy.

## TECHNIQUE OF ADMINISTRATION

In order to obtain good therapeutic results from ECT and to minimize possible complications, the following are important guidelines to follow prior to, during and after ECT:

1. Carefully assess the patient's health by taking complete history and doing physical work-ups with emphasis on cardiac and neurologic problems.

2.   Medical consultation should be obtained prior to ECT in any patient whose psychiatric illness is complicated by serious or unstable medical condition (e.g., cardiac failure or arrhythmia, uncontrolled diabetes mellitus, myxedema, etc.). The psychiatrist should then weigh the consultant's opinion along with all the other factors to be considered in making the final decision for or against ECT (4).

3.   C.B.C., U.A., chemistry, VDRL, chest, skull and dorsal spine x-rays, EKG and EEG should be considered. If neurological is abnormal, CAT is important.

4.   Consent for treatment is obtained. The patient must be informed about the treatment he will receive. The task force of the American Psychiatric Association suggests giving the patient a description of the treatment before he signs a consent.

5.   Advise the patient not to eat or drink for at least four hours prior to the treatment (to avoid vomiting and aspiration).

6.   All psychotropic drugs should be omitted on the morning of the treatment.

7.   Nausea can be avoided with 100 mg dimenhydrinate (Dramamine®) prior to the treatment or IM after the treatment, or prochlorperazine 5 mg. IM prior to the treatment or IV after the treatment (5).

8.   Atropine, given in a dose of at least 0.6 mg subcutaneously, IM or IV is most commonly used (it will decrease the morbidity of the treatment due to both cardiac arrhythmias produced by vagal stimulation and aspiration due to excessive production of saliva during and after the seizure). Since atropine is an agent that acts centrally in addition to systematically, it may increase confusion following the treatment, so the APA task force on ECT recommended the use of methylscopolamine which does not cross the blood brain barrier.

9.   The patient should be encouraged to empty bowels and bladder prior to the treatment.

10.   Artificial dentures should be removed.

11.   Loose teeth should be extracted (they may break and be aspirated during the seizure).

12.   In order to prevent the patient biting his tongue or lips during the convulsion, a gauze-covered tongue depressor or mouth gag should be inserted between the upper and lower teeth (3).

13.   Prior to ECT, the patient is anesthesized with an ultra short-acting barbiturate, in most cases methohexitol sodium

(Brevital®) I.V., approximately 1 mg/kg body weight. Brevital® is less cardiotoxic and has more rapid action than the older thiopental sodium (4). We give Brevital® to avoid the psychological distress related to placement of electrodes and other activities directly prior to ECT and the physical discomfort related to the muscle relaxant that is given to prevent fracture, dislocations, muscle pain and exhaustion.

14. A neuromuscular depolarizing agent, succinylcholine (Anectine®) is given to produce muscular relaxation or to suppress strong muscular contraction and avoid fractures and dislocations. The convulsive activity need not be completely suppressed unless the patient has severe musculoskeletal pathology. The administration of succinylcholine may result in prolonged apnea as a result of a congenital deficiency of the enzyme pseudo-cholinesterase. The succinylcholine is given rapidly I.V. after the onset of anesthesia. Empirically determined dose of succinylcholine is chosen (30-80 mg) that will block the strong muscular contractions.

15. One hundred percent oxygen is begun per bag.

16. The neck is extended through upward traction on the chin.

17. Patient's temples should be cleansed with alcohol sponges before treatment to eliminate cutaneous sebun and because it may adhere to electrodes and increase electrodes' own resistance, which may cause inadequate response or even skin burns (3).

18. Metal electrodes should be coated with conductive jelly; cloth-covered electrodes should be wetted with saline.

19. Both electrodes should be placed in the anterior portion of the temples (bilateral placement or treatment), but in order to mitigate possible dysmnesia and confusion unilateral treatment should be used (6, 7, 8), placing the temporal electrode on the bisection of a line that connects the outer corner of the eye and the beginning of the pinna of the ear over the hemisphere non-dominant for language (right hemisphere in 95% of the patients) and the second electrode is held about three inches above the first one directly toward the vertex.

20. Electric current should be applied in strict accordance with the directions for the particular machine being used. The effective seizure-inducing stimulus range is 140 to 170 volts for 0.5 to 1.0 seconds. While it is quite possible to obtain seizures at settings below 140 volts for 0.5 seconds, the proportion of missed

or incomplete seizures (subconvulsive stimuli) is significantly increased, frequently resulting in the need for a second application of current and resultant loss of the advantage of the initial lower-energy impulse. It is advisable to use the lowest setting which will consistently induce general seizure in the individual patient being treated (4). The electric current is an alternating current. The amount of current applied to the head during the stimulation has a maximum of 1600 miliampers. The ordinary electrically induced convulsion if not premedicated is characterized by a tonic phase followed by clonic movements which in the beginning are fast and of small range, and later become slower and more forceful until they fade out after a total of 30–50 seconds for the whole seizure. The convulsion is accompanied by apnea. The patient may lose urine, semen or seldom, feces (5). Safe ECT requires adequate preseizure and postseizure oxygenization with 95–100% oxygen.


## RISKS AND COMPLICATIONS

In general, the risks and/or complications from ECT are less than when patients are treated with drug therapy. The complications related to ECT can be divided into morbidity and mortality. Statistics show that mortality associated with ECT has been about 1 per 10,000 patients, and deaths have been generally attributable to cardiac complications (9).

*Morbidity of ECT.* Prior to the use of muscle relaxants, the most frequent complications of ECT were fractures and subluxations compression fractures of the dorsal and mid-thoracic spine between T4 and T8, but since the introduction of succinylcholine, they are relatively rare.

*Cardiovascular complications.* The most serious complications related to the cardiovascular tree are: cardiac arrhythmias, cardiac arrest and myocardial infarction, the two latter complications occurring almost exclusively in individuals with pre-existing cardiac disease (3). The most common type of cardiac complications are premature ventricular contractions mediated to vagal hyperactivity, with onset usually during brief postictal bradycardia. The use of atropine or methylscopolamine has generally alleviated this problem (10).

*Neurological.* Aside from symptoms of aggravation of brain tumors, neurological complications are extremely rare.

*Prolonged apnea.* This is usually associated with the prolongation of succinylcholine's muscle relaxant effect, generally resulting from a congenital relative deficiency of the enzyme pseudocholinesterase.

*Postconvulsive excitement or emergence delirium.* The patient is agitated, restless, assaultive, unreasonable. This state lasts for about 10–15 minutes and can be terminated with phenothiazines IM or diazepam 10 mg I.V. This condition is rare.

*Nausea and vomiting.* This can be prevented with dimenhydrinate and prochlorperazine IM before or after ECT.

*Headache.* Post seizure headache occurs in about one third of the patients, and usually is relieved by aspirin or acetaminophen.

*Amnesia.* The amnesia can be retrograde and anterograde, depending on a number of factors:

1. With unilateral ECT, the memory is disrupted less than with bilateral ECT (4, 11).
2. The degree of amnesia varies with the type of psychopathology. Amnesia is usually less in nondepressed patients, particularly in schizophrenic patients who may be resistant to the amnesic effects of the seizures (11).
3. Performance and memory tasks decay with each successive seizure during the course of the treatment.
4. Currents of high intensity disrupt memory the most. When ECT is given with certain drugs, the memory impairment could be accentuated, i.e., lithium (12), l-tryptophan (13); or decreased, i.e., amphetamines (14) or pemoline (15).
5. Memory and recall prior to the illness recover completely, while memory of events that occurred during the treatment or related to the immediate pretreatment period may be lost permanently.
6. The severity of memory loss may be modified by maximum spacing of treatments (11).

*Electrode burns.* These may occur when there is not a uniform conduction due to irregular pasting of the electrodes (in bilateral ECT) or putting the electrodes too close together when using unilateral treatment.

*EEG changes.* They have been found to occur after ECT, but seem largely transient. They consist of 3-6 cups moderately high voltage slow waves. These waves usually disappear in a period of three weeks to three months. Most of the time, these waves appear after six to eight treatments.

## HOW ECT WORKS

Nobody knows exactly how ECT relieves the symptoms of the psychiatric problems it is indicated for, but cerebral biogenic amine activity increases after one seizure, and persists after four to six seizures (16). The release of hypothalmic peptides, as prolactin and ACTH, is increased with seizures. Also, it has been found in animals that ECT produces a decrease in the sensitivity of the postsynaptic B–noradrenergic receptors. This is due either totally or in part to a decrease in the density of the B–adrenergic receptors (17). ECT also appears to produce a sustained increase in synthesis and utilization of NE and increase of dopamine and serotonin turnover (1).

## NEUROPATHOLOGY

Reports of human material in regard to possible damage from ECT in the brain are scarce. New investigations confirm the early findings by Alexander & Lowenbach that even stimulation lasting several seconds causes only reversible changes caused by vascular mechanisms and that currents of shorter duration as used in ECT do not lead to recognizable findings. Experiments in animals show evidence that ECT produces no important morphological changes in the brain (11).

## USE OF ECT

*General indications.* ECT should be the physician's initial preference when:
1. Previous episodes of the same illness have not responded to drug treatment.

2. The patient's medical condition (first trimester of pregnancy, history of multiple drug allergies) makes drug use inadvisable.
3. When the patient's illness is severe and progressing so rapidly that no time is available for even a brief trial on drugs.
4. The available treatment facilities are inadequate or the responsible family members cannot be relied on to supervise his medication (3).

## SPECIFIC INDICATIONS

1. Psychotic depressions
2. Catatonic state
3. Manic phase of bipolar disorder
4. Schizophrenias that are unresponsive to drug therapy.

ECT shows marked efficacy in depressions, mainly in major depression, unipolar or bipolar depression, depressions with psychotic features and depressions with melancholia. Seriously depressed patients should be treated with ECT when there is a danger of suicide, when they don't respond to antidepressants, if they become severely withdrawn, profoundly anoretic or if they have a sleep disorder which is getting worse. Secondary but still valid indications are: manic episodes which don't respond to either lithium or neuroleptics, catatonia (stuporous or excited) when the patient appears to be dangerous to himself and those around him and cannot be controlled with drugs, schizophrenias that are unresponsive to other therapies. The more acute the schizophrenic disorder, the better the response to ECT. Other disorders have been treated with ECT, but except for the conditions mentioned above, the treatment has not been very successful (10).

## CONTRAINDICATIONS

There are no absolute medical contraindications for ECT (4). In patients with serious medical liabilities, it is necessary to modify the ECT procedure but treatments can be given. In some textbooks, intracranial pressure or brain tumors are considered an absolute contraindication (1,3,18); excluding the rare need for ECT in such a patient, there are records of successful ECT even in these conditions of very high risk. In addition, there are many other medical conditions in which ECT should only be considered and given with consideration for the special precautions that would improve the safety of the treatment. Patients with cardiac pacemakers may be treated safely.

## CONDITIONS OF SPECIAL CONSIDERATION FOR ECT

| *Symptom* | *Complication* |
| --- | --- |
| Increased intracranial pressure | Cerebral & vascular hypertension |
| Recent myocardial infarction | Vascular hypotension, cardiac failure |
| Cardiac arrhythmia | Exaggerated arrhythmia |
| Porphyria | Barbiturate toxicity |
| Recent fracture | Fracture |
| Liver disease, malnutrition | Low cholinesterase activity |
| Organic mental disorders | Organic psychosis confusion |
| Glaucoma | Acular hypotension with atropine |

## FREQUENCY AND DURATION OF TREATMENT

Clinicians differ in their views regarding the total number of treatments needed in a particular illness. Usually ECT is given three times a week. Treatment should be continued until symptoms are well relieved. Most of the time, this occurs after six or eight treatments, usually from 12–20 seizures are given to the patients. Behavioral criteria is used principally to determine the number of treatments. A therapeutic window may be developed in the future based on the number of seconds or total seizure time. Maletsky suggested between 210 and 600 seconds of total seizure time may be optimal for a course in patients with depressive psychosis. Fewer than 12 to 20 treatments are rarely successful in schizophrenia (11). Multiple seizures have been used in rapid succession in the past.

Outpatient ECT can be administered to nonhospitalized patients but close supervision from a responsible person is very important. Such a person should receive instructions in regard to insuring the patient has nothing by mouth for about 12 hours before ECT, accompanying the patient from treatment, and closely supervising the patient for at least four hours following the treatment.

## THE USE OF ECT AND DRUGS

It has not been proven that the simultaneous use of psychotropic drugs and ECT has any advantages.

Neuroleptic drugs are hypotensive and mention has been made of some hypotensive complications in patients under ECT when chlorpromazine is added. The danger is definitely greater with rauwolfia drugs, which should be discontinued. This latter drug may increase the incident of cardiac arrhythmias and cardiac arrest (19). Many people avoid giving the patient neuroleptic medication on the morning of the treatment; others avoid the combination all together.

Lithium should not be co–administered with ECT as it may prolong the neuromuscular blockade with succinylcholine (20). For the same reason, antibiotics such as streptomycin and related compounds should also be avoided. There is also a report of severe organic confusional state occurring after combined therapy with ECT and lithium (21).

## COMPARISON OF ECT
## AND PSYCHOTROPIC MEDICATION

Due to different problems, including nosological distinctions between schizophrenias and affective disorders, interpretations of investigations, dose of medication, duration of the treatments and other factors that may affect the most carefully designed study, it has at times been difficult to reach a sound conclusion when ECT has been compared to psychotropic drugs. In spite of these problems, certain conclusions seem apparent. For severe depression, ECT is reported to be superior to antidepressants (22).

## CONCLUSIONS

More research is necessary in order to understand the reasons why ECT works.

## REFERENCES

1. Salzman C: Electroconvulsive therapy. In: Shader RI (ed), Manual of Psychiatric Therapeutics. Boston: Little, Brown and Company, 1975.

2. Kurland AA, Hanlon TE, Esquibel AJ, Krantz JC Jr, Sheets CS: Comparative study of hexafluorodiethyl ether (Indoklon®) and electroconvulsive therapy. J Nerv & Ment Dis, 129:95, 1959.

3. Detre T, Jarecki H (eds): Modern Psychiatric Treatment. Philadelphia: J.B. Lippincott Co., 1971.

4. Abrams R, Essman W (eds): Electroconvulsive Therapy: Biological Foundations and Clinical Applications. New York: S.P. Medical and Scientific Books, 1982.

5. Kalinowsky LB, Hippius H, Klein HE (eds): Biological Treatments in Psychiatry. New York: Grune and Stratton, 1982.

6. Goldman D: Brief-stimulus electric shock therapy. J Nerv Dis, 110: 36-45, 1949.

7. Cannicott SM: Technique of unilateral electroconvulsive therapy. American Journal of Psychiatry, 120:477-480, 1963.

8. Lancaster NP, Steinert RR, Frost I: Unilateral electroconvulsive therapy, J Ment Sci, 104:221-227, 1958.

9. Fink M: Efficiency and safety of induced seizures (ECT) in man. Comp Psychiatry, 19:1-18, 1978.

10. Weiner RD: The psychiatric use of electrically induced seizures. American Journal of Psychiatry, 136:1507-1515, 1979.

11. Fink M: Convulsive Therapy: Theory & Practice. New York: Raven Press, 1979.

12. Small JG, Kellams JJ, Milstein V, Small IF: Lithium in combination with ECT — possible negative interactions. Personal communication in Fink M (ed) Convulsive Therapy: Theory & Practice. New York: Raven Press, 1979.

13. d'Elia G. Lehmann J, Raotma H: Influence of memory functions in depressive patients treated with unilateral ECT. Acta Psychiatric Scand, 57: 259-268, 1978.

14. Mah CJ, Albert DJ: Reversal of ECT-induced amnesia by post ECT injections of amphetamines. Pharmacol Biochem Behav, 3:1-5, 1975.

15. Small IF, Sharpley P, Small JG: Influence of Bylert upon memory changes with ECT. Amer J Psychiatry, 125:837-840, 1968.

16. Fink M: Neuroendocrine Aspects of Convulsive Therapy. In Abraham R, Essman W (eds), Electroconvulsive Therapy: Biological Foundations and Clinical Applications. New Yori: S.P. Medical and Scientific Books, 1982.

17. Mendel J, Amsterdam JD (eds): The Psychobiology of Affective Disorders. New York: S. Krager, 1980.

18. Kolb LC, Brodie HKH (eds): Modern Clinical Psychiatry, Tenth Edition. Philadelphis: W.B. Saunders, Co., 1982.

19. Bracha S, Hes J: Deaths occurring during combined reserpine-electroshock treatment. American Journal of Psychiatry, 113:25, 1956.

20. Jefferson JW, Creist JH: Primer of Lithium Therapy. Baltimore: Williams & Wilkins, 1977.

21. Small JG, Kellams JJ, Milstein V, Small IF: Complications with electroconvulsive treatment combined with lithium. Biol Psychia, 15:103-112, 1980.

22. Siris CS, Glassman AH, Stener F: ECT and psychotropic medication in the treatment of depression and schizophrenia. In Abraham R and Essman WB (eds), Electroconvulsive Therapy: Biological Foundations and Clinical Application. New York: S.P. Medical & Scientific Books, 1982.

# Chapter 13

## BASIC MENTAL HEALTH NURSING SKILLS

LOIS C. FRIEDMAN, Ph.D.
BEVERLY HEBERT, B.S., R.N.

What are mental health nursing skills? By whom are they practiced, when, and in what settings? How can they be learned, and how can they be integrated with other aspects of nursing practice? In this chapter, we will deal with these, and similar, questions in an attempt ot define what we mean by "mental health nursing" and to demonstrate that these skills are essential to good patient care in all areas of nursing practice, not simply in the single specialized field of psychiatric nursing.

What we mean by "mental health nursing" is not the same as what usually is meant by psychiatric nursing. Psychiatric nursing is that branch of nursing practice which deals with the care of psychiatric patients, whether as inpatients or outpatients; and is a specialty of the nursing profession, just as are pediatric nursing, obstetrical nursing, surgical nursing, and so on. Mental health nursing, on the other hand, enters into all nursing specialties; and although mental health nursing skills definitely are required in psychiatric nursing, they also are essential in pediatricians' and obstetricians' offices, labor and delivery suites, and operating and recovery rooms, if the nursing practice in these, as in other, settings is to be good nursing.

Essential to our concept of mental health nursing is a focus on health rather than on pathology or illness. This distinction frequently is overlooked in discussions of psychiatric nursing (1). Lack of attention to the difference, and to its implications, may have the effect of severely limiting nurses' effectiveness. An emphasis upon personality pathology may alienate patients who do not wish to be identified as psychiatrically ill. Unfortunately, the notion of pathology frequently is conveyed by well-meaning but poorly informed nurses who deal with patients in non-psychiatric contexts. It is this attitude of caring for psychiatrically ill patients that we wish to dispel.

First, however, we must define what we mean by mental health nursing. Mental health nursing may be thought of as including *all those behaviors engaged in by nursing personnel which are specifically directed toward meeting the psychological and emotional needs of patients and patients' families.* Mental health nursing skills, therefore, are of paramount importance in psychiatric nursing. However, what we mean by mental health nursing is both more and less than what is implied by psychiatric nursing: more, because mental health nursing enters into *every* nursing specialty; less, because some of psychiatric nursing (for example, meeting patients' physical needs, or administering medication) is not primarily intended to meet patients' emotional needs, although the way in which such tasks are carried out may or may not do so. Mental health nursing also differs from psychiatric nursing in the assumption of health which is basic to a philosophy of mental health. People with psychological and emotional needs are not necessarily psychologically or emotionally ill. The fact that all of us have such needs means that helping to meet them is part of maintaining or restoring health, rather than treating illness. This assumption — that people are fundamentally healthy — is central to the attitude underlying all mental health nursing.

In the remainder of this chapter, we will consider the following: What are the fundamental skills involved in mental health nursing; where and when are these skills practiced; how can they be learned; and how can they be integrated into traditional aspects of nurses' roles, such as the nursing process.

## FUNDAMENTAL MENTAL HEALTH NURSING SKILLS

The skills basic to effective mental health nursing have much in common with the elements of effective helping relationships in general. The latter have been identified by Truax and Carhuff (2) as *accurate empathy, nonpossessive warmth,* and *genuineness.* Research has demonstrated that these three traits are characteristic of effective psychotherapists regardless of their theories, personalities, and patient populations. Furthermore, these ingredients of helping relationships are interdependent; in order to have an empathetic understanding of the experiences and feelings of others, one must also have a feeling of warmth for them; and for one's warmth and empathy to be meaningful to others, one must be perceived as being genuine, authentic, or "real."

In order to achieve the goals of genuineness and empathy, nurses' interactions with patients must be characterized by an absence of defensiveness. This necessitates that they be aware of and sensitive to their own personality dynamics, especially areas of intrapersonal conflict which have not adequately been resolved. Similarly, the expression of nonpossessiveness warmth requires an understanding of one's own needs, in order to prevent these from interfering with one's ability to recognize and meet the needs of patients. As is true for all helping relationships, care must be taken to avoid using other persons (e.g., patients) to satisfy one's own needs, lest this satisfaction take priority over the most basic reason for the existence of the relationship, that is, the provision of assistance.

For example, nurses with strong needs to be liked unconsciously may keep patients recovering from surgery from expressing their anger at those upon whom they are dependent. Consequently, these patients may turn their unexpressed anger inward and experience intensified feelings of depression. Such situations might be avoided if nurses were aware of the psychological discomfort which they feel when dealing with patients' anger, and if they were able to encourage patients to express these feelings, as well as others which often lie behind, and may be concealed by, the angry ones. Similarly, nurses who have particular difficulty dealing with death, faced with patients who have been diagnosed as having terminal illnesses and who nevertheless are continuing to behave cheerfully, may accept superficially bright affect as being indicative of the absence of depression, rather than considering the possibility that these patients either are denying their fear of death or are avoiding discussing it because of the anxiety which it arouses in others.


## THE WHEN AND WHERE
## OF MENTAL HEALTH NURSING

Ideally, the fundamental concepts and skills of mental health nursing should be an integral part of all nursing practice. In actuality, however, the integration of psychological principles into nursing care often proves more difficult. Nurses and nursing administrators frequently become preoccupied with the more routine aspects of nursing care; and patients' physical needs typically are accorded a higher priority than their emotional needs, in part because nurses often feel more comfortable and competent dealing with the former than the latter. What sometimes is not recognized, however, is that routine nursing procedures also offer opportunities for nurse–patient interaction, and are potential vehicles for the exercise of mental health nursing skills. Furthermore, since some requests for physical care are really an expression of, and an attempt to call attention to, patients' emotional and psychological needs, the application of mental health nursing skills actually may reduce the number and/or urgency of patients' demands, thereby making nurses' workloads lighter rather than heavier. The contention that nurses do not have sufficient time or energy to attend to their patients' mental as well as physical health needs fails to take into account this relationship between the two kinds of patient needs, and eventually may contribute to nurse "burnout."

In addition to the practice of mental health nursing skills leading to an eventual expansion of available time because of the consequent reduction in patients' demands, nurses are in a unique position to recognize, assess, and meet patients' psychological and emotional needs because they provide care on an around-the-clock basis. They observe patients at all times of day, in contrast to physicians, whose observations are limited to small samples of time (often at the same time of day, each day, as well); and they see patients under a variety of conditions and circumstances, observing their reactions to different events and occurrences, both expected and unexpected. Nurses frequently are also the first (and last) members of the health care team who patients see as they enter and leave the hospital or office; and sometimes nurses are the only contact patients have with the health care system, such as in public health nursing, industrial nursing, and school health nursing.

The answer to the question of when mental health nursing skills should be utilized is simply, "always." Nurses (and, for that matter, all health professionals) never should overlook the potential psychological importance of all interactions with patients, no matter how non-psychologically-oriented such interactions may appear to be. In addition to this, nurses are in a position of particular importance with regard to recognizing and responding to patients' emotional needs, since they are not only the first and last people to see patients, but also are the only ones who observe and care for patients continually, including at those times (such as the middle of the night) when patients' defenses may be lowest and their emotional needs most evident.

The answer to the "where" of mental health nursing is most emphatically, "everywhere." As we stated at the outset, mental health nursing skills should not be confined to psychiatric settings. In fact, it is probably in nonpsychiatric settings that patients' mental helath needs are greatest, because it is there that they are overlooked most often. This includes both outpatient and inpatient facilities; and not only settings such as patients' rooms, but settings such as x-ray departments and operating and recovery room as well.

Mental health nursing skills are not acquired automatically, nor are they learned easily. Furthermore, the skills discussed in this chapter are not sufficient without a thorough foundation in the psychology of personality and psychopathology. In particular, nurses need to be familiar with the different kinds of psychological defense mechanisms (denial, projection, reaction formation, and so on); theories of personality, and how different personality types characteristically react in different kinds of situations; and the nature of human behavior when people are subjected to physical and emotional stress. A background in developmental psychology is desirable also, since the fear and pain experienced by many patients may produce regressions to earlier stages of maturation; and a knowledge of the different stages of personality development may help nurses both understand what is happening when this occurs, and assist patients in working through the crises and regaining their previous (or even higher) levels of maturation.

Three other sources of learning are important for the acquisition of mental health skills as well. These are: modeling; supervision; and personal growth and self-understanding (i.e., insight). By "modeling" is meant the imitation of role models, that is, persons whose behaviors one wishes to acquire. Modeling goes hand-in-hand with supervision; as students begin to practice the behaviors of their role models, supervisors are needed to assess and comment upon (give "feedback" about) the students' performance. Although nursing students usually have a plentiful supply of role-models available during their training, it is important that these be selected for specific purposes. It is possible that good role-models for learning mental health nursing skills might not be nurses at all, but rather people from other mental health-related disciplines. In fact, one could suggest that non-nruses should be included among those persons who assess students' mental health skills, on the basis that outsiders to nursing are less likely to be distracted by details of nursing practice unrelated to the exercise of mental health skills, and may be better able to focus exclusively on nursing students' exercise of these skills as a result.

Finally, good mental health nursing requires an understanding of oneself and a willingness to look at one's reactions to, and interactions with, different kinds of patients. Although people vary in their degree of insightfulness, the greatest degree of insight is obtained through participation in psychotherapy, either individual or group. Nursing is a career which makes heavy emotional demands upon those who choose it; and, as Moffic and Gomez (3) point out, "there seems to be a strong relationship between the emotional status and effectiveness of the caregiver." These authors advocate some form of personal therapy for mental health professionals for the purpose of dealing with their own resolved conflicts, as well as for dealing with the stresses generated by being in caregiver roles; and the incorporation of this idea into nursing education and training (on a voluntary basis, of course) would be a valuable addition to any program designed to teach fundamental mental health nursing skills, whether to nursing students or to veteran nurses.

## MENTAL HEALTH NURSING SKILLS
## AND THE NURSING PROCESS

The common denominator and *sine qua non* of all branches of nursing is the *nursing process:* a dynamic problem-solving technique consisting of the four phases of assessment, planning, intervention, and evaluation (4). The first phase, that of *assessment*, involves the collection of data (biological, psychological, and social) about patients. This includes information regarding both present and past behavior, as well as events that are current in patients' lives, and past events that continue to hold significance for them. The next phase, *planning*, involves the development of a blueprint for the nursing intervention. This includes identifying patients' needs (nursing diagnoses) and writing nursing care plans. Nursing care plans state the nursing goals; how the goals will be reached (the nursing actions); and what outcomes are expected to result from the actions (1). The *intervention* phase is the actual implementation of nursing plans. It is during this phase that nursing care is coordinated with the contributions of other health care personnel. The final, *evaluation*, phase is the measurement of the effectiveness of the nursing actions. During the evaluation phase, the initial assessments of patients' needs are reviewed, along with the nursing care plans and the outcomes of the interventions. In actual practice, this last phase is integrated with the preceding three phases, rather than coming at the end of the process; as new information is learned, or patients' needs change, the original assessments are reviewed and nursing care plans are adjusted accordingly.

The interface between the nursing process just described, and the basic mental health nursing skills discussed earlier, occurs in the exercise of two additional skills which are fundamental not only to mental health nursing, but to all aspects of nursing practice. These are *observation* and *communication*. The observant nurse is alert to all aspects of patients' behavior that may reflect their psychological or emotional states: facial expression; voice quality; dress and grooming; posture; mood and affect; perceptions; thought processes; cognitive functioning; and interpersonal relationships (including response to other patients, staff, and family members). Without good observation skills, neither the first (assessment) nor the fourth (evaluation) phases of the nursing process could be carried out; and in the absence of good assessment and evaluation, the information needed for the other two (planning and intervention) phases would not be available.

The process of observation, furthermore, is intertwined with, and dependent upon, that of communication. Nursing observations are not a one-way process. Complete and accurate observations of human behavior require interacting with the people who are being observed; and it is only through a two-way process of communication with patients that nurses are able to check the accuracy of their initial observations (assessment) and determine the efficacy of their interventions (evaluation).

Understanding the elements of effective communication is as important as the other fundamental skills discussed here in terms of the importance of their contribution to good mental health nursing. Communication occurs on both verbal and nonverbal levels, and begins the very first moment that nurses and patients meet. The initial rapport which nurses establish (or fail to establish) with patients may persist for the duration of their contact with each other, ranging from single office visits to entire hospitalizations or even years or decades that patients remain in the care of their physicians and the nurses whom they employ. The establishment of this rapport (which includes encouraging patients to express their thoughts and feelings freely and openly) is facilitated by the exercise of the three basic mental health nursing skills: genuineness, warmth, and empathy. What nurses say (or fail to say), how they say it, how well they listen, and how they act — each of these influences whether patients trust nurses sufficiently to "open up" and communicate to them what they need to know in order to do their jobs effectively.

Once initial rapport has been established with patients, nurses need to continue the communication process, so that the flow of information will not be impeded. One way of doing this is by taking a "nondirective" approach (reflecting back to patients what they have said and emphasizing the feeling aspects rather than the specific content). Hopefully, this will have the effect of making patients feel understood thereby, encouraging them to continue expressing themselves. Again, the qualities of being warm, genuine, and emphathetic may make the difference between success and failure in this regard.

What specific things can nurses do to project these qualities in such a way that they are perceived by patients? Both verbal and non-verbal behaviors are important. Such verbal behaviors as using patients' names, allowing patients to set the pace and tone of conversations, asking patients to clarify what is unclear, restating what patients have said, and checking out with patients how well they really are understood — all of these communicate positive impressions to patients. Verbal behaviors which should be avoided generally include being (or sounding) judgmental, giving one's own personal opinions, giving false reassurances, engaging in monologues, and barraging the patient with questions. Non-verbal ways of conveying positive impressions include sitting near patients, looking directly at them, and giving them one's undivided attention (1). For both verbal and non-verbal behaviors, receiving supervision is important; and if this is not available, nurses may want to work in pairs occasionally, alternating in adopting the "practitioner" and "observer" roles so that all of them receive feedback on their performance from the others. Of course, these specific behaviors will be effective only to the extent that the people exercising them really feel the qualities which they are trying to convey; and nurses who find it difficult or impossible to feel genuine, warm or empathetic a significant amount of the time are urged to seek professional assistance. Some hospitals now employ part or full time trained nurse counselors to assist nurses with their own mental health problems.

## SUMMARY

We have presented the fundamental mental health nursing skills which can and should be practiced by nurses from all specialties and in all settings. Mental health nursing differs from psychiatric nursing in its emphasis upon health rather than upon illness, and by the way in which it enters into every branch of nursing practice, non-psychiatric as well as psychiatric. Mental health nursing includes "all those behaviors engaged in by nurses which are specifically directed toward meeting the psychological and emotional needs of their patients and their patients' families;" and the three fundamental skills of mental health nursing are *accurate empathy*, *nonpossessive warmth*, and *genuineness*. Since patients' demands for physical care frequently are indications of unmet psychological needs, the small amount of extra time required to pay attention to patients' emotional states will more than "pay for itself" in terms of greater patient satisfaction and less nurse exhaustion.

Although these three fundamental skills are not practiced exclusively by nurses, nurses are in a unique position to recognize and meet patients' emotional needs, because they alone provide care on an around-the-clock basis. Furthermore, nurses frequently are the first and last (and sometimes are the only) health professionals whom patients see. Nurses also integrate the contributions of other members of the health care team. The effective exercise of mental health nursing skills, therefore, is basic to good patient care.

The four phases of the nursing process (assessment, planning, intervention, and evaluation) have been described; and the interface of the nursing process with the practice of mental health nursing was discussed in terms of nurses' abilities to observe and communicate. Effective nurses put their mental health skills (empathy, warmth, and genuineness) to use in the nursing process; through the exercise of observation and communication and the more emphathetic, warm, and genuine they are, the better will be their observation of, and communication with, patients. Nurses need to be aware that they communicate non-verbally as well as verbally. Communication is a two-way process, the goal being the creation of an atmosphere of trust, so that patients will feel free to share their thoughts and feelings with nurses. The success of this depends in part upon the initial rapport which nurses establish with patients; and the tone of these initial contacts is likely to last for the entire time that patients remain in treatment.

The ways in which nurses can acquire these basic mental health nursing skills include having good role-models; receiving supervision directed specifically at the exercise of these skills; increasing their knowledge of human behavior through formal coursework in such areas as personality, abnormal, and developmental psychology; and gaining greater personal insight and stability so that their own roles in various kinds of nurse-patient interactions will be more therapeutic. In this regard, nurses should consider entering into some form of psychotherapy, either individual or group, as part of their training; the objective of this being to increase their insight and self-awareness, and to resolve their unresolved psychological conflicts, so that they will be more effective in helping other people to deal with their own emotional and psychological difficulties. In these and other ways, the practice of fundamental mental health nursing skills results not only in improved patient care, but also in increased satisfaction and personal meaning to be derived from the profession of nursing.

## REFERENCES

1. Taylor CM: Mereness' Essentials of Psychiatric Nursing, 11th Ed. St. Louis: C.V. Mosby Company, 1982.

2. Truax CB, Carhuff RR: Toward Effective Counseling and Psychotherapy: Training and Practice. Chicago: Aldine Publishing Company, 1967.

3. Moffic HS, Gomez EA: Personal treatment for the mental health caregiver. In Moffic HS and Adams GL (eds), A Clinician's Manual on Mental Health Care: A Multidisciplinary Approach. California: Addison-Wesley Publishing, Company, 1982.

4. Schaefer J: The interrelatedness of decision making and the nursing process. American Journal of Nursing, 74:10, 1974.

# Chapter 14

MANAGING THE SOCIAL SYSTEM

JOAN BROCHSTEIN, M.S.W., M.P.H.

In years past, health and mental health problems were generally diagnosed and treated in a simple, straightforward manner. That is, if parents brought their child to a psychotherapist claiming that he was a trouble maker or a problem child, the therapist would in all likelihood evaluate and treat the youngster for the complaint made by the parents and investigate no further. Similarly, if a patient approached a physician about headaches, the doctor would most likely inquire no deeper into the problem than to take a medical history and do a diagnostic workup, considering the patient's problem on strictly physical grounds.

Fortunately, this rather narrow approach to health and mental health care is diminishing and increasingly being replaced by a perspective which judges the presenting problem within the context of the patient's life situation and takes into account the many factors which might cause or contribute to the profession for a great many years and which is now coming into favor in health and mental health facilities across the country (1).

This philosophy, known to the social work community as the person-in-situation gestalt or configuration, is the basis of all professional interventions made by the provider (2). Essentially, this approach is to look beyond the presenting problem to the context in which it occurs so that the patient's complaint is not seen as an isolated issue in his life. The provider looks to the effect of the social network on the patient's health and symptoms and on the prognosis of treatment. He considers all the factors which impinge on the patient's health and seeks to understand the patient in light of interpersonal, cultural and socioeconomic factors which affect him. As it becomes increasingly clear to providers the enormous power that the environment has in shaping the person and how one's health, physical and emotional, are linked to his life situation, the more the professional is interested in "treating" the context as well as the individual.

The stress that exists in one's life circumstances, whether it be financial, occupational or family problems, can lead to physical and emotional difficulties which bring the individual into the health professional's sphere. Once the patient has sought help from such an individual, the problem is often seen simply as a physical or emotional problem and is treated as such. When this is the case, the underlying problems are overlooked while the symptoms may be treated quite vigorously. Such an approach may provide temporary relief to the individual, but unfortunately will not address the real issues at hand.

In the case of mental health care, it is unlikely that a troubled individual can make significant strides in treatment if the stresses in his life are profound and a matter of survival (3). Thus, a woman may seek help for depression and she in fact may have a number of symptoms of a clinical depression, i.e., loss of appetite, crying spells, sleep difficulties, and so forth. A traditional mode of treatment would be to treat her with antidepressant medications or to perhaps initiate long-term psychoanalytically-oriented psychotherapy to get at the causes of her depression. In fact, one or both of these treatment choices may be appropriate if the reality of the woman's situation so dictates. But all too often the external factors in the patient's life are overlooked and their importance discounted as significant causative factors in her depression. If, for example, she is a single parent with a low paying job, and many problems to contend with, her pain and difficulty in functioning may be appropriate to the circumstances of her life. Addressing the reality of her life situation by exploring possible changes in her environment may be far more reasonable as a treatment approach than traditional means of treating depression, at least at the outset. Once the financial pressures are eased or her daycare problems remedied, the depressive symptoms may lift.

When the patient is facing life-threatening circumstances, such as lack of food or the inability to pay for heat in the dead of winter, the exploration of psychological issues is of virtually no value. A precept of quality mental care is  to acknowledge and respect a patient's readiness for psychological work. This means that a therapist will not push the patient to explore or understand issues which he is not ready to face; it also means, simply, that if a person is confronted with the loss of employment, all insight as to why he has lost yet another job is worthless in the face of his financial worries. If the individual has no means of feeding his children and paying his rent, the therapist would be ill-advised to spend valuable therapeutic time on the psychological issues underlying the patient's predicament. More vital at this time is helping the person to handle the concrete steps which he must take to stabilize his life situation. Once the family is fed and cared for and the individual has a reliable job once again, the intrapsychic issues can be addressed.

How the therapist proceeds with a new patient depends on the severity or immediacy of the situation and upon the resources available to the individual or his capacity for taking steps on his behalf. Although the initial phase of therapy may focus on helping the patient to deal with external problems, the goal of the therapist is always to move beyond this point to working with the patient to develop his general level of functioning and quality of life.

Any effective form of treatment, whether it is crisis intervention or long-term psychotherapy, must work with the individual's environment to some degree. The milieu in which one lives, the general parameters of one's life, have great impact on the individual's frame of mind and the expectations that he has for himself and his family. It is incumbent upon the practitioner to fully investigate with the patient the social stresses in his life, past and present, in order to gain full understanding of the person's circumstances. This relates to general environmental influences such as the individual's ethnic background and way of life as well as to specific areas such as income and housing. The goals and the prognosis of treatment all are interwoven with the external realities of the patient's life. According to the person-in-situation approach to treatment, the individual and his environment are seen as an interdependent, interacting balance of forces, each influencing the other (4). The practitioner must seek to separate and identify these inter-connecting forces in order to understand the environmental factors which affect the patient and his family, to understand the individual's personal dynamics and his relationship with family members, and very significantly, to understand the way in which the patient views and reacts to his environment. The individual interacts with his environment on two planes: the everyday external factors that he must confront (e.g., heavy traffic or family arguments), and the effect that these problems have on his emotional life and equilibrium.

External influences are generally internalized by the individual to a very great extent. His view of the world, hostile or trusting, and his concept of his own worth are closely connected with his social environment. The value system which he lives by, his attitudes and behavior patterns and even the kinds of health and mental health problems he develops are all heavily influenced by the external forces to which he is exposed.

The way in which a therapist works with a patient, the mode of treatment which he chooses, depends to a large degree on his understanding of the person/situation continuum and the forces affecting the individual — psychological, social, economic. The provider must be finely attuned to these environmental influences if he is to grasp the essence of his patient's life situation. A comprehensive and integrated assessment plays a pivotal role in bringing about such an understanding of the patient and his problems.


## ASSESSMENT

Early contacts between patient and clinician constitute the diagnostic and assessment phase, or consultation phsse, of treatment. It is during this time that the clinician gains a sense of what the problems are and what factors are instrumental in causing these difficulties. It is also the time to formulate a treatment plan for the patient and, if appropriate, for his family.

Before the clinician makes any judgments as to the nature of the patient's problem, it is essential that he take into consideration all pertinent aspects of the patient's life circumstances. In forming an opinion as to the person's ability to function, the therapist must have an adequate picture of the pressures operating in the individual's life. The general background of his life situation — the social and cultural makeup of his community, neighborhood conditions, educational and vocational opportunities available — are all broad areas of understanding which the practitioner should have as a backdrop for understanding the subtle influences in the patient's life.

On a more concrete level, the therapist needs to acquire basic information on the person's circumstances — whether there is economic hardship, who lives in his household, what sort of job he holds, what, if any, religious affiliation he has, how his physical health is. The quality of the relationships in his life is of paramount concern — whether he is an isolate or is surrounded by family and friends. How he relates to others in his social network — employer, co-workers, teachers, peers, neighbors — is important information for the therapist to learn during this consultation phase. Additionally, the developmental milestones in the person's life, the quality of his childhood, the basic dynamics in his family of origin, and the history of the presenting problem must come under scrutiny if the therapist is to fully understand the patient's needs.

Overall, the clinician's purpose during the assessment process is to attain a general sense of who the patient is, his needs and desires, his strengths and limitations. Much of this he should be able to elicit from the patient, unless there are reasons why the patient is not equipped or willing to work with the therapist. Often, however, it is necessary or advisable to explore these questions with collateral contacts, with family members or other significant persons in the patient's social network. In some cases, as with multi-problem families, the practitioner may have to seek information from the records of other agencies with which the family has been involved.

## FAMILY EVALUATION

The decision as to whether to involve family members in the diagnostic process is generally based on the clinician's early impressions of the patient, his presenting problem and the meaning of the problem to significant others in the patient's life. If it appears that the family could be helpful in providing insight or perspective into the patient's difficulties, or, more importantly, if it seems likely that the problem is serving some function for the family as a whole, it is likely that the therapist will want other family members to participate in the assessment process, and often in the treatment itself (5).

The question of what possible function a family member's symptoms might serve for the family as a whole is often a source of puzzlement for those not acquainted with family therapy theory. According to students of family therapy, a family member may become labelled as the one in the family with a problem, while in contrast all other family members seem to be normal and healthy. The "identified patient" is in a sense scapegoated and blamed for the family's difficulties and the family feels that all of their problems reside in this one individual. Family theorists believe that the symptoms or troubled behavior manifested by a given individual should be seen as a reflection of a dysfunctional system of which he is a part (6, 7). The disturbed behavior of one member is essentially a form of communication to his family and to others that he, and indeed the family as a whole, are in trouble and in pain. The problems which appear in one family member are seen in terms of personal and interpersonal conflict and also as reflecting a process which runs through the entire family (8). The family often unconsciously supports the identified patient's deviant behavior in order to maintain a sense of balance and predictability in the family (9); by focusing on the problems of one family member, the family is able to mask and overlook other, perhaps even more painful, problems in the family. The delinquent behavior of an adolescent boy or the school refusal syndrome of the latency–aged girl may occupy the family's attention while other more profound difficulties are hidden from view, such as the crumbling of the parents' marriage, or an incestuous relationship between the father and daughter. In a sense, the child's problem serves as a protective function for the family by deflecting attention from severe problems that the family does not want to acknowledge.

The question of whether or not to interview other family members is clearcut in certain cases, and a matter of the therapist's opinion in others. When the identified patient is unable to speak for himself — in cases where he is retarded or severely emotionally disturbed, or if the patient is a child, the therapist will need to rely on information reported by others. In this kind of assessment, the identified patient has most likely been involved with schools and other agencies or medical programs, and the information acquired from these facilities will also be significant in coming to a diagnosis and treatment plant.

In those cases where engaging family members in the assessment process would be detrimental to the patient, contact with the family should be avoided. This would occur when meeting with the family would be of no particular value in the evaluation and would perhaps jeopardize the relationship between the patient and his therapist. If there is no suspicion on the part of the practitioner that the patient's symptoms are related to family conflicts and problems, there is no valid reason to engage the family in the process.

When it does appear to the therapist, however, that there is family dysfunction and that the patient is the "carrier" of the family's problems, it makes good sense to meet with the whole family in order to view the problems in the interpersonal arena in which it occurs (10, 11). By arranging for one or more family interviews, the therapist has the opportunity to observe family dynamics firsthand and to gain direct knowledge of the system in which the patient's symptoms developed and are being maintained. In a family session, roles, alliances, and conflicts between family members can be seen as interactional patterns and family attitudes and beliefs come into focus. The focus of power and control, issues of dependency and autonomy, and the general level of functioning can be ascertained through direct observation of the interaction between family members. By noting the verbal exchanges as well as body gestures, seating patterns and other non–verbal cues, the therapist is able to determine rather quickly the nature of the problem and the position which the identified patient holds in the family.

Although family members often initially resist any interpretation of the family's situation which might relieve the identified patient of his scapegoat role and which might redefine the source of the problem, it is generally the case that the presenting problem gives way to a different definition of the family's problem. It is not uncommon to bring to light pain or conflict involving other family members which previously went unnoticed or unmentioned in the family.

In determining who should be included in the family assessment, it is appropriate for the therapist to bring in anyone who has an emotionally significant relationship to the patient. This would include his immediate family but may also include his girlfriend, extended family members, even employers, teachers, or neighbors. In order to determine the meaning of the symptoms to the patient and his family, conjoint interviews with all appropriate individuals may be supplemented by meetings with subgroups (e.g., the patient's parents or the patient and his spouse) or by interviews with other individuals in the family system.

Engaging family members in the assessment process must be managed with great care and sensitivity by the therapist in order to develop and preserve the delicate balance with his patient(s). Confidentiality must be maintained at all times, so that those interviewed can feel free to disclose their true feelings and concerns. It is essential that all contacts with family members be above board and with no air of secrecy or manipulation. Here the skill of the therapist is of utmost importance, for a good working alliance with several family members is difficult to achieve. The therapist must be aware of the potential conflicts which can arise, and he must be attuned to the feelings and needs of all concerned so as to facilitate the process.

Through sensitive and careful interviewing, the therapist, in a relatively brief span of time, should be able to formulate a comprehensive and basically accurate picture of the patient's condition. He should be conversant with the patient's life situation to the extent that he can determine whether the present difficulties are due to psychological factors or a dysfunctional system and whether changes are necessary within the person or his environment or both. If the therapist determines that environmental factors play a pivotal role in the individual's problems, his focus will most likely be on treating or modifying those factors rather than focusing on intrapsychic issues in the patient. If it appears that family conflicts are at issue and are the basis for the patient's symptoms, the therapist will be inclined to work on changing the family system rather than working with the patient individually. If, on the other hand, it appears that intrapsychic issues must be addressed, then the therapist will, in all likelihood, recommend individual therapy.

Overall, the purpose of the assessment process is to reveal the individual's or family's needs, where the source of the problem lies and what resources are available to correct the problem. Identifying the sources of stress, be they external or internal to the individual, is of utmost importance. It is important to discover why the patient's coping mechanisms failed at this time, what was the precipitating stress which led to his loss of equilibrium. The patient's current level of adaptation, the dynamics of his present life and recurrent behavior patterns should be examined in relation to his background and life experiences.

The plan of treatment recommended by the therapist is a natural outgrowth of the findings which emerged in the assessment process. By exploring both the internal and external factors impinging on the individual and their meaning in his life, the therapist views the patient with full regard for his situation and is able to come to a dynamic understanding of the patient's difficulties.

## TREATMENT

Based upon his findings during the consultation phase, the therapist makes his determination as to the best course of action. He should at this point have a clear sense of the external stresses operating in the individual's life and the patient's ability to cope with these difficulties. He should have a feel for the patient's overall functioning and ego strength and an understanding of the nature of the problems and how they fit in the patient's life. If the family is heavily invested in the symptoms of the individual and his problems are symptomatic of family pain, it is likely that the therapist will want to engage the family in treatment rather than limiting therapy to the identified patient. If not, the therapist will proceed with the person on an individual basis.

When the practitioner believes that the patient is not capable of handling the stress in his life on his own, and particularly if the problems are external in nature, i.e., housing or employment problems, the therapist may feel that he must take an active and directive stance initially. That is, he may help the individual with specific ideas and plans so that the patient can begin to stabilize his situation. The therapist might take on this active role in instances where the person is severely depressed and immobilized, has limited intellectual abilities, or has impaired reality testing. Likewise, if the patient simply does not have the necessary energy or personal resources available and has no support system, the practitioner would be likely to step in.

The therapist makes interventions on the patient's behalf and plays an active role in solving the patient's difficulties at the risk of furthering the individual's dependency needs and sheltering the patient from growing up and handling his own affairs. It is obvious, therefore, that being directive is a tactic which is done selectively and as infrequently as possible. When it is necessary to use this appropach to get the patient on the road to taking responsibility for his problems, it is an acceptable practice (12). But the therapist's intent should always be to help the patient become more and more willing and capable of solving his own problems, initially with the support of the therapist, and eventually on his own or with the help of his own personal support system.

Interventions made by the therapist on the patient's behalf should be seen by both parties as an interim measure until the patient is able to do such things on his own. If at all possible, the therapist should act as an ally and as a catalyst to the patient, enabling the individual to take on as much responsibility as he can.

The kinds of interventions which the practitioner may engage in might include contacting a financial assistance agency or a health clinic to insure that the patient obtains needed assistance, arranging for job training or legal advice, hiring a housekeeping service, or calling the school for a child in the family who is failing. If the patient is functional, none of this would be appropriate for the therapist to do. But, if the patient is overwhelmed and is struggling with an unmanageable life situation, the therapist's interventions can relieve some of the strain and enable him to regain a sense of equilibrium. Once a kind of balance is established, the possibility of looking at the underlying issues and causes of the problems may occur. In any case, stabilization of the external situation is a necessary step in the treatment process.

If the patient is able to function but is confused and unable to make decisions, the role of the therapist is still directive but less involved than when the patient is immobilized. In this instance the therapist may make concrete suggestions to the patient and support him in carrying out the suggestions. Thus, rather than on the one extreme calling an agency for the patient, or on the other extreme helping the patient to realize that he should call the agency, the therapist will specifically recommend to the patient that he call the particular agency. He may, in fact, provide the individual with the name of a contact person, the phone number and other pertinent information in order to ease the process for the patient.

Regardless of the stage the patient is in — partly functional or unable to function at all — the therapist's goal is to help the patient to become as self-directed and resourceful as possible so that he will not need to depend on others. Helping the patient to develop his coping skills and to attain a sense of control in his life are primary concerns of the therapist. By modeling new ways for the patient to perceive and act on the stresses in his life, the therapist helps the individual to gain a sense of mastery and to learn how to problem-solve (13). By learning to identify and clarify the issues that trouble him, the patient can begin to develop ways to change the things in his life which distress him, to plan a course of action and to predict the results of his action. Inasmuch as possible, the therapist refrains from telling the patient what to do but provides a climate in which the patient can test out various ideas and feelings without risk. The therapist's objectivity, coupled with his commitment and interest in the patient, are of enormous value to the patient who is at a loss and in need of guidance. By helping the patient to correct his own distortions and misperceptions, the therapist can enable him to let go of self-imposed pressures and to develop a more realistic view of what is possible and how to attain it (14).

If the therapist has decided to take a family-based approach to treatment and is working with the identified patient and appropriate family members, the principles of developing the family's problem-solving capacities and ability to handle their difficulties apply as well. The distortions and communication pitfalls which occur in troubled families are addressed, as the source of the real problem comes into focus. As in the case of working just with an individual patient, the therapist is interested in developing awareness and clarity on the part of the family members so that each person takes responsibility for his or her own actions, feelings and decisions. In this way the scapegoating behavior that occurs in the family is no longer needed and the family becomes free to change and grow.

Whatever the focus of the therapeutic work, be it individual or family-oriented treatment, the relationship between external and internal issues in the patient's life is always a prominent feature. The therapist keeps in mind the bearing which the environment has on the individual's inner world and conversely, the way in which the individuals' psychological makeup contributes to the course of his life and the environment in which he lives. The practitioner makes use of the every day problems of the patient in order to help him to develop psychological insights into his difficulties. By gaining mastery over the small difficulties he encounters on a day-to-day basis, the patient eventually begins to feel a sense of control and authority in his life generally. In learning to perceive and to relate more clearly to these dilemmas and problems, the individual can understand and modify his usual, possibly dysfunctional, modes of behavior and replace them with ways which work and enable him to feel happier and more successful. As he is able to incorporate these new approaches into his life as a whole, new possibilities in life open up and eventually the support of the therapist is no longer needed.

## CONCLUSION

The profound influence of the individual's life situation on his mental health is increasingly being regarded as a vital and necessary area of inquiry by psychotherapists. To disregard the effects of poverty, stressful family relations or unfulfilling employment on the individual's ability to function is to do one's therapeutic work in a vacuum. Working with environmental issues is a pivotal aspect of psychotherapy, for the individual's intrapsychic problems are closely interrelated with the difficulties and stresses of his everyday life. By addressing even the most mundane problems, the patient can begin to deal with patterns and conflicts which affect his well-being and the choices he makes in life. Although the therapist cannot hope to work on deep intrapsychic issues with a patient who is experiencing severe environmental stress, it is possible, as therapy proceeds, to artfully weave the work of psychotherapy into the realities of everyday living. Psychotherapists who fully appreciate and utilize the stresses in their patients' lives in their work, are far more effective than those who overlook those issues and move quickly to intrapsychic issues without orienting themselves to the cultural and socioeconomic milieu in which patients live. For therapy to work the whole of a patient's life situation must be explored. By looking through a wide lens into the individual's life, the therapist can discover who the patient is in all his complexities. This is the cornerstone of effective psychotherapy.

# REFERENCES

1. Brochstein JR, Adams GL, Tristan MP and Cheney CC: Social Work and Primary Care: An Integrative Approach. Social Work in Health Care, Vol. 5(1):71–81, Fall, 1979.

2. Hamilton GH: Theory and Practice of Social Case Work. New York: Columbia University Press, 1940, 1951.

3. Brochstein JR: The Environment in Evaluation and Treatment. In Moffic HS and Adams GL (Eds), A Clinician's Manual on Mental Health Care: A multidisciplinary Approach. Menlo Park, California: Addison Wesley Publishing Co., 1982, pp. 120–127.

4. Hollis F: Casework: A Psychosocial Therapy. New York: Random House, 1972.

5. Brochstein JR: "Families and Interpersonal Social Systems in Evaluation and Treatment." In Moffic HS and Adams GL (Eds), A Clinician's Manual on Mental Health Care: A Multidisciplinary Approach. Menlo Park, California: Addison Wesley Publishing, 1982, pp. 110–119.

6. Bowen M: The use of family therapy in clinical practice. Compr Psychiat, 7:345–374, 1966.

7. Satir V: Conjoint Family Therapy. Palo Alto: Science and Behavior Books, 1964.

8. Stamm IL: Family Therapy in Casework: A Psychosocial Therapy. Edited by F. Hollis. New York: Random House, 1972.

9. Jackson DD: The Question of Family Homeostasis. Psychiatric Quarterly Suppl, 31:79–90, 1959.

10. Haley J: Family Therapy. In Freedman, Kaplan and Sadock (Eds) Comprehensive Textbook of Psychiatry, 2nd edition. Baltimore: Williams and Wilkins, pp. 1881–1885.

11. Jackson DD, and Satir V: A review of psychiatric developments in family diagnosis and family therapy. In Ackerman NW, Beatmen FL and Sherman SN (Eds), Exploring the Base for Family Therapy. New York: Family Service Association of America, 1961.

12. Taber LR: Social Work: A Basic Service. In Fink AE (Ed.) The Field of Social Work. New York: Reinhart & Winston, Inc., 1974.

13. Perlman HH: Social Casework: A Problem–Solving Process. Chicago: University of Chicago Press, 1957.

14. Friedlander WA (Ed.): Concepts and Methods of Social Work: Englewood Cliffs, NJ: Prentice Hall, 1976.

# Chapter 15

## HOW TO REFER AND TO WHOM

### TIMOTHY L. BAYER, M.D.

Suggesting that a patient seek psychiatric care can be very uncomfortable for health care professionals. They can appreciate in part the patient's feelings about the referral and in fact, may exaggerate these feelings in their own mind. They are likely to be uncertain about how the patient will react and the effect that this intervention will have on their working relationship with him. They are likely to feel concerned that their suggestions may prove hurtful to the patient. They may have some doubts themselves about the usefulness of psychiatric treatment. They don't know how to sort out the various mental health professionals providing services and to decide which one would be best for this individual. And, if they have waded through all of these concerns, they often don't know what to say to the patient. Despite this discomfort, most health care professionals who have direct contact with patients are likely at some time to encounter patients who they feel are in need of mental health care.

## HOW PATIENTS FEEL ABOUT PSYCHIATRIC REFERRAL

Several studies have attempted to evaluate just how patients respond to being referred for psychiatric treatment. Koran, *et al.* (1) investigated the way hospitalized patients react to a referral to a psychiatrist. They interviewed a group of patients after being seen by the psychiatrist. When initially seen, 72% of the patients had an accepting and cooperative attitude toward the referral. Among those who had a mixed or negative attitude toward referral initially, more than half of them felt afterwards that the consultation with the psychiatrist had been helpful. Of all the patients, 63% found the consultation very helpful, while 20% believed that it had been of little or of no value. Half of the patients who had negative attitudes were substance abusers. The authors of this study feel that a significant factor leading to the generally positive response to referral in these patients was the way they were prepared during the referral process.

Despite the generally positive response to referral shown in this study, there are a number of patients sho display negative responses. In another study by Hale and Abram (2), 17% of the patients felt offended or angry when told that a psychiatrist would be coming to see them. These studies suggest that while the majority of patients will respond favorably to referrals, it will be important to explore with patients any negative feelings or fears they may have regarding a referral.

Another concern health professionals may have regarding a referral is whether the referral will alter their ability to work with the patient. Will the patient's opinion about the referring professional change? Schwab, *et al.* (3) asked a number of patients referred to psychiatrists by their doctors whether the referral had changed their opinions about the doctors. Seventy percent stated that the referral had not changed their opinions at all. Most of the subjects who did express a changed opinion felt that the referral increased their respect for their doctor and was often seen as evidence of his concern for them.

## WHY PATIENTS MAY FEEL RESISTANCE
## TO PSYCHIATRIC REFERRAL

*"What will people think of me?"* "Do you think I'm crazy?" Despite some changes in attitudes toward the mentally ill during the last half century there is still some stigma attached to mental illness and to seeking psychiatric care. The mentally ill are often seen as bad people rather than as suffering people. Schwab (4) noted that patients' tendencies to be influenced by these negative views are in part determined by the attitudes of the hospital staff. When the patient is referred, he is likely to be particularly sensitive to the attitudes of the person making the referral. He will be testing out the general reactions he is likely to encounter from others by evaluating the attitudes of the medical staff as they discuss the referral. He is likely to ask either in subtle or direct ways, "Are you sending me to this person because you don't like me or

want to get rid of me?" When discussing the referral, it will be important to be alert for these concerns. The patient needs to hear that he is not being abandoned or thought of as bad.

*"Will the psychiatrist read my mind?"* "Will he want to talk about things I don't want anyone to  know?" Some of these concerns refer to what Schwab (5) has called the mystique of psychiatry. Mental health workers are seen as having special, mysterious powers and abilities. In addition, these concerns relate to anxiety about entering a relationship in which uncomfortable thoughts and feelings are discussed. Patients often have little understanding of how psychotherapy works or what the therapist will do. They are anxious about what kind of person the therapist will be and what he will think of them. It is important that the person who discusses the referral have some knowledge of what takes place in mental health treatment. He should be alert to concerns the patient has regarding the nature of the treatment and regarding the psychotherapeutic relationship.

*"Can anyone really help me?"* Much of the work in demonstrating the effectiveness of psychiatric treatment is still in progress. Studies testing the effectiveness of psychiatric treatment are often difficult to do. Patients are likely to have doubts about how much can actually be done for them. Yet, there is evidence for the effectiveness of various treatments including the psychotherapeutic techniques and medications. Part of the patient's concern may also relate to the feelings of hopelessness that accompany many forms of mental illness. These feelings are particularly common in depressed patients.

It is important when discussing referrals, to impart a sense of hopefulness and to address the patient's hopelessness. It is useful to point out to the patient that certain forms of mental illness are often accompanied by a sense that nothing will help. Patients also often feel that they do not deserve to be helped. The patient should be told that these feelings are a part of what will be addressed in the treatment.

In addition, the person discussing the referral needs to have a basic knowledge of just what psychiatric treatment can and cannot do. He should know what problems respond best to treatment. He needs to be able to give hopeful but realistic information to the patient regarding what can be accomplished.

*"Will talking about my problems make them worse? I'm holding on as tight as I can?"* Although patients will not always say these sort of things, they are likely to have a sense that talking about their problems or changing their behavior will only make things worse. Many of the manifestations of mental illness are thought to represent, in part, attempts at coping with very difficult situations. But these attempts at coping are made in maladaptive ways. The patient, in a sense, is doing the best he can given his circumstances and background. Part of treatment involves finding new mechanisms for coping. Because this means giving up the old mechanisms, many patients are likely to fear giving up something that may have prevented further decompensation.

The person discussing the referral also needs to attend to these concernes. Judgmental statments are likely to make the patient want to defend his behavior even more. It is generally better to acknowledge the fact that the patient seems to have tried his best in coping with his difficulties, but that perhaps it would be useful to discuss other ways of handling the situation. Most forms of psychiatric treatment allow patients to gain further control over their lives. They are not forced to do things against their will. The patient should be reassured that he will be helped to make changes in his life, but only when he feels ready to do so.

*"What will the treatment cost?"* "Will I finish treatment not only unhappy but also broke?" In fact, psychiatric treatment can involve some expense to the patient. The availability of psychiatric coverage in health insurance tends to be variable and many health insurance policies cover half or less of the cost of outpatient psychotherapy. Issues of payment are often important in the therapeutic process and some therapists have suggested that patients respond better when they are given the opportunity to contribute financially to their treatment. Studies examining the use of other health services by people who receive psychiatric treatment (6) have suggested that in fact, patients who receive psychiatric treatment are less likely to be in need of other expensive medical treatment. This may be partially due to the fact that people who do not receive psychiatric treatment are likely to seek help for their problems through other medical services.

The patient who has limited financial resources should still be able to receive competent psychiatric care. Most communities have clinics which are funded either by the government or by charitable organizations which offer mental health care for a fee which is based on the patient's income.

## WHERE TO REFER: WHO DOES WHAT

There are a number of mental health resources available and it often becomes difficult to sort out which type of service will best fit the needs of a particular patient. There are also a variety of mental health professionals providing services. There tends to be some overlap in what each professional does but there are also some differences in terms of services provided, the approaches to treatment and the training that each individual has received. The three major providers of mental health care are psychiatrists, psychologists, and social workers.

*Psychiatrists* are physicians who have received specialty training in psychiatry after completing medical school. This specialty training usually consists of a three to four year residency program during which the trainee receives experience in both inpatient and outpatient treatment. Psychiatrists are able to prescribe medication and administer electric shock treatment. Also because of their general medical training they are particularly able to evaluate for medical illnesses which might lead to mental changes. They also receive training in psychotherapy and may be experienced in working with individuals, groups, or families. They may either work individually or in association with other mental health professionals. Therefore, it is possible that they will either treat patients themselves entirely or only be involved with some of the treatment while receiving assistance from other mental health workers. All psychiatrists must be licensed for the practice of medicine in the state in which they practice. Many psychiatrists are also certified by the American Board of Psychiatry and Neurology, an organization which evaluates the training which the psychiatrist has received and administers an oral and written examination to further evaluate for competency.

*Clinical psychologists* have generally received a doctoral degree (Ph.D.), although in some areas persons with master's or other degrees can be called psychologists or psychological associates. In addition to their advanced university training, they also generally are required to complete an internship of approximately one year which consists of practical clinical experience in addition to the clinical and academic experience they have gotten in their earlier training. They are particularly skilled in administering diagnostic tests but also receive training and experience in individual, family, and group psychotherapy. Laws regarding licensing and registration tend to vary from state to state. There is a standard examination used in evaluating who may be licensed. They may practice on their own but they are often likely to be associated with other professionals. Many psychologists have physicians available for consultation and treatment with medication if this should be necessary. Psychologists who are diplomates in the American Board of Professional Psychology have met standardized requirements for training and experience and have successfully passed a written and oral examination.

*Social workers* have generally received a master's degree in social work (M.S.W.). Doctoral programs in social work are also offered by some schools. Bachelor's degrees in social work are also available, although people with these degrees generally function with some supervision. Not all social workers have received direct training in psychotherapy and social workers sometimes specialize in areas such as administration and in social agency case work. Social workers generally have special competence in assisting patients in their interactions with various social agencies. Many social workers are also particularly trained in evaluating and treating families. Laws regulating the practice of social workers also vary from state to state. In some areas social workers may practice on their own but very often they practice in association with other mental health professionals. Social workers may be members of the Academy of Certified Social Workers (ACSW). In order to qualify for membership in this organization, a social worker must hold a master's degree in social work, must have completed two years of experience in an agency while under the supervision of a member of the ACSW and must have completed a national examination.

*Nurses* seldom practice individually but are often part of mental health care teams. Some large hospitals have nurse clinicians available to other nursing personnel for assistance in managing difficult patients. Nurses function in mental health services in a variety of capacities. They administer and supervise the use of medications but also may be involved in individual, group, or family psychotherapy.

*Counselors and ministers* vary widely in the amount of training they have received. They tend to have little experience in evaluating or treating the more severe forms of mental illness but may be particularly experienced in dealing with marital and family problems.


## HOW TO LOCATE A REFERRAL

Mental health services also vary widely in terms of services provided, types of problems treated and fee arrangements.


### Patients in Hospitals

Many general hospitals have psychiatric consultation/liaison services. Other hospitals have psychiatrists available on their staff to provide consultation. The consultation/liaison service will provide evaluation of patients with psychiatric problems, particularly those patients whose emotional problems interfere with medical managements. They generally work with a medical team in developing a treatment plan. They will be available to the health care professionals in providing suggestions for the optimal management of difficult patients. They are also available for assistance in arranging for referrals to outpatient services when the patient is ready for discharge.

Psychiatric consultations are usually done at the request of the treating physician, and the decision to seek consultation should be discussed by the medical team. Most consultation/liaison services are also willing to informally discuss patient management problems and to provide education regarding psychiatric illness.

Some hospitals also have nurse clinicians available to assist nursing staff in the management of difficult patients. They generally do not see the patient in a formal way, but are available to the staff for discussion of the problems being encountered with the patient.


### Outpatients

Some outpatient clinics also have psychiatric consultation services available. It is generally useful to maintain contact with some mental health profession who can give advice on referral sources. If such resources are not available, there are a number of ways to locate referral sources.

*Community mental health centers* are available in many areas. They can provide a wide range of mental health services. They are generally available for evaluation and can also provide referrals to other facilities. Many of these centers have received support from the federal government. In order to qualify for this support, centers are required to provide certain essential services including inpatient, outpatient and emergency care. They are required to be available to offer assistance to other health care professionals in locating referral sources.

*Private practitioners* may either practice individually or in groups. Generally they are willing to discuss the types of problems they prefer to manage and will refer to other practitioners those patients they cannot or prefer not to manage.

*Local mental health organizations* are also available in many communities. They can provide information regarding the various services available within the community.

*Educational institutions*, particularly those which have training programs for mental health workers, often maintain patient care facilities which see patients at reduced fees. They often also maintain lists of practitioners in the community who are available for outpatient referrals.

*Local medical societies* will provide lists of physicians who meet minimum licensing requirements within the area and are available for new patient referrals.


## Patients Who Require Psychiatric Hospitalization

Patients who are thought to be dangerous either to themselves or to others often require hospitalization. Other patients may also be hospitalized in order to receive evaluation, observation, or treatment which might not be available to them as outpatients.

State laws govern the ways that patients can enter and remain in mental hospitals. There are basically two legal conditions under which patients can enter a mental hospital.

*Voluntary admissions* occur when the patient understands and agrees with the need for hospitalization. The patient retains all of his legal rights. He may choose to leave the hospital at will although some states allow the hospital to hold him for a specified time to arrange for involuntary hospitalization if his doctors feel it would not be safe for him to leave.

*Involuntary admissions* (commitment) occur when the patient is judged to be both:

1.  Suffering from a mental illness which requires hospitalization (usually because of danger to the patient himself or to others), and,

2.  unable to appreciate the need for hospitalization.

In some states, this is a legal decision and patients are committed by a judge who listens to the testimony of physicians and concerned family or friends. In other states, this is a medical decision and patients may be held after being examined by a specified number of physicians. In these states, the patient then has the right to a legal hearing but does not automatically receive one unless he requests it. The committed patient has lost his right to decide whether to stay in the hospital, but this does not necessarily mean that he has lost his other civil rights. Unless the courts say otherwise, he may maintain his rights to do such things as voting and managing his other personal and financial affairs.

Most mental health professionals can provide information regarding the admission procedures in a given state. They can also assist in evaluating the need for hospitalization.

## WHO NEEDS A REFERRAL

Studies which have examined the prevalence of mental illness in the community have suggested that a large percentage of the population may be suffering from some form of mental illness. Two well-known studies have looked at the prevalence of mental illness in individual communities. The Stirling County Study (7) looked at the entire population over age 18 in a rural county in Nova Scotia. Twenty percent of the population were found to have a disorder which interferred with their lives severely enough to require clinical attention. The Midtown Study (8) looked at a sample of the people between ages 20 and 59 living in midtown Manhattan. In this study, 23.4% of the sample were thought to have symptoms severe enough to produce serious impairment. On the other hand, the study of Hollingshead and Redlich (9) looked at the number of people in the town of New Haven who were actually receiving mental health treatment. They found the prevalence of treated persons to be less than 1%. More recent estimates (10) suggest that the current percentage of the population in treatment may be closer to 1.5%–2.0%. These studies suggest that many people suffer from symptoms severe enough to impair their functioning but that few of them are currently receiving treatment for these symptoms. The reasons why so few people receive care probably include the patients' concerns mentioned previously. Currently, mental health services would be unable to adequately care for the large number of potential patients identified in these studies. Many of these people are likely to seek assistance from other medical services.

The decision regarding which patient then requires referral needs to be based on considerations regarding both the patient and the health care team. Some patients can be effectively managed within a medical setting. Both basic psychotherapy and medications can often be provided by health care professionals who have knowledge of basic treatment techniques. It is important that all persons providing care to these patients know their limitations and consider referral when these limitations are reached.

In addition, several factors regarding the patient need to be considered. A basic knowledge of the psychiatric diagnosis is important and attempts should be made to at least consider the diagnostic possibilities suggested by the patient's problem. Knowledge of which problems are most likely to respond to treatment can then be applied to the referral decision. Consideration should also be given to the extent that the patient's symptoms have interferred with his functioning. Questions about difficulties with performing at work should always be asked. All patients should be encouraged to discuss the nature of their relationship with family members and other important people in their lives. Often, emotional disorders interfere with medical management and many of these patients can also benefit from some psychological intervention.

Thus, the decision to refer needs to be based on the nature and extent of the problem, the degree to which the problem interferes with areas of functioning, and the availability of other resources to the patient.

Although these guidelines allow for some flexibility, there is one group of patients who always require special attention. Patients who are thought to be at risk for suicide either because of recent suicide attempts or because of thoughts or plans regarding suicide should always receive full evaluation.

## WHAT TO SAY TO THE PATIENTS

Very often, one of the more important tasks in discussing a psychiatric referral with the patient, is not what is said but what the patient is given an opportunity to say. It is important to allow ample time to discuss the patient's concerns and to clarify any misconceptions that he may have. So-called "shotgun reassurance" based on hunches regarding the patient's concerns are rarely as useful as reassurance based on a clear understanding of the concerns the patient has expressed. Thus, throughout the discussion the patient should be given frequent encouragement to voice his concerns and his reactions to what is being said.

The discussion regarding referral should generally begin with a clear statement of the psychological problems that have been identified. It is generally useful to emphasize the statements that the patient has made about his problem, and the reasons why these statements indicate a need for further help with the problem. The patient should be told some of the positive aspects of receiving treatment for these problems. It should be made clear that the referral is not being made because the medical team has been unable to find anything wrong with the patient or feels that they have nothing further to offer him. Instead, the patient should be told that psychiatric evaluation will be useful in providing further assistance to him. Patients who feel abandoned by the medical team or who feel that they are being sent to the psychiatrist as a last resort are often less cooperative with psychiatric treatment.

After discussing the nature of the problem and the reason why the problem suggests the need for mental health care, the patient should be given some information regarding what can be expected from psychiatric evaluation and treatment. It is generally important to inquire about previous treatments and discuss any reactions the patient might have had to the previous treatment or other contact with mental health professionals. The patient should then be told about where he is being referred. In some cases, it will be necessary to present several of the treatment settings available to him and discuss differences in terms of fees and psychotherapeutic approaches, giving the patient an opportunity to assist in the planning for the referral. Near the end of the discussion, the patient should be given a final opportunity to express any feelings or concerns about the referral. Special attention should be paid to evidence that the patient has distorted in some way what has been said. If these distortions can be clarified, the patient is far more likely to cooperate in the referral.

Referral sources should be asked in advance whether they prefer to be contacted by the patient himself or by the referring health care professional. Unlike other health care providers, many mental health care services prefer that patients arrange for appointments themselves. It is, therefore, important to insure that the patient fully understands the procedure for obtaining an appointment.

The decision regarding who should discuss the referral with the patient is generally one that should be made by the medical team as a whole. Most often, the person primarily responsible for the patient's management should discuss the referral directly with the patient. However, patients will frequently ask other members of the health care team questions regarding the referral. Other staff members should be available to listen to concerns that the patient may have and to either reassure the patient or refer him back to the person who has done the original discussion.

Most mental health workers who have received referrals from health care professionals are aware of the importance of what the patient is told. They know that further compliance with treatment will be in part determined by the way that the patient has been prepared. They will generally be willing to discuss any problem which might arise in presenting a referral to the patient.


## CONCLUSION

Despite concerns to the contrary, many patients quite readily accept referrals to mental health services. The process of making the referral can be made more comfortable by being sensitive to the patient's feelings and concerns regarding the referral. Knowledge about the resources available and the indications for treatment will make the discussion easier. The discussion with the patient should then include a factual, nonjudgmental description of why the treatment is indicated and how, where, and with whom it will occur. Patients need to be given adequate opportunities to express their reaction to what they have been told.


## REFERENCES


1. Koran LM, Van Natta J, Stephens JR, *et al.*: Patients' reactions to psychiatric consultation. JAMA, 241:1603-1605, 1979.

2. Hale ML, Abram HS: Patients' attitudes toward psychiatric consultations in the general hospital. Va Med Mon, 94:342-347, 1967.

3. Schwab W, Clemmons RS, Valder MV, *et al.*: Medical patients' reactions to referring physicians after psychiatric consultation. JAMA, 195:1120-1122, 1966.

4. Schwab JJ: Handbook of Psychiatric Consultation. New York: Appleton-Century-Crofts, 1968.

5. Schwab JJ: Consultation from the psychiatrist. In Usdin G and Lewis JM (Eds.), Psychiatry in General Medical Practice. New York: McGraw-Hill, 1979.

6. Mumford E, Schlesinger HJ, Glass GV: The effects of psychological intervention on recovery from surgery and heart attacks: an analysis of the literature. Am J Public Health 72:151-151, 1982.

7. Leighton DC, Harding JS, Macklin DB, *et al.*: The Character of Danger: The Stirling County Study, Vol. 3. New York: Basic Books, 1963.

8. Langner TS, Michael ST: Life Stress and Mental Health, Thomas AC Rennie Series in Social Psychiatry, Vol. 2. New York: Free Press of Glencoe, 1963.

9. Hollingshead A, Redlich FC: Social Class and Mental Illness. New York: Wiley, 1958.

10. Breiser M: Psychiatric epidemiology. In Nicholi AM (Ed.), The Harvard Guide to Modern Psychiatry. Cambridge: The Belknap Press to Harvard University Press, 1978.

# Chapter 16

## THE MENTAL HEALTH CHECK-UP:
## A LOOK AT PREVENTION

### H. STEVEN MOFFIC, M.D.

*"An ounce of prevention is worth a pound of cure."*
*Anonymous*

Potentially, almost anybody involved in human services is in the position to do a mental health check-up (1). However, allied health and nursing professionals have special opportunities in this area which can be utilized for the health of their patients. With their role of caregivers, such professionals are in a privileged position to hear about potential mental health problems and to exert a therapeutic influence themselves or via referral to others. This is not to say that health providers should be intrusive into patients' personal lives, not to go beyond the strict guidelines of their work, but rather to be sensitive and open to hearing about psychological issues which so often arise in the context of health problems.

The mental health check-up can be thought to consist of two related dimensions (2). One conception is that mental health is the absence of mental illness. In this conception, the basic role of the health professional in a check-up would be to look for early signs of mental disorders. The other conception is that mental health can be promoted and enhanced in its own right. Here we are dealing with the ability of individuals to reach their psychological potential.

Within this framework, a check-up could be incorporated into a variety of health care activities. A patient could reveal significant fears during blood-drawing; or, a patient with cancer would be directed to using the rest of their life in the most useful manner. The important point here is how stress is handled, not whether stress is present or absent.

In other words, prevention can be considered to be any activity designed to decrease the development of mental disorders or that will lead to enhanced mental health. For instance, a nurse doing pregnancy care could help to identify parents who may otherwise later neglect and abuse their children. This nurse could also help in providing parenting information which would increase the satisfaction of being parents. In the mental health sense, prevention is like good nutrition. Good nutrition generally enhances your physical status and development, while at the same time it can help to prevent some later health problems. Or one could use the metaphor of successful military or football strategy: a good offense is the best defense. Strengthening the person or reducing undue reactions to stress is the offense here.

Although primary prevention has long had a solid theoretical and practical basis (3), it nevertheless still is not a major activity in the mental health field. Both the stigma of mental illness and the need to treat significant suffering have helped to limit primary prevention activities. However, the concerned health practitioner will still have ample opportunity to practice some sort of primary prevention. The mental health check-up provides one model and attitude for such activity. The mental health check-up is based on the well known periodic health examination, the physical check-up. Unfortunately, a mental evaluation has not yet become a routine part of the physical check-up.

## WHAT TO LOOK FOR

The basic opportunity for allied health and nursing professionals to apply the mental health check-up is as part of their routine activities. A view toward assessing the reaction to the stress the patient is experiencing will lead to appreciation of various warning signs which may signify the beginning of some kind of mental disorder. Several isolated symptoms should be noted by any alert health practitioner.

### Change in Sleep Patterns

Sleep is often the most sensitive measure of a person's mental well-being. While different people have different routine needs for sleep, a change in the usual pattern often indicates the presence of emotional stress. Usually, there is a reduction of sleep, but there can also be an increase. In addition, a change in dreams, especially the presence of nightmares, can be important clues for undue stress. Any health professional worker working the night shift in hospitals can readily pick up such changes, and other practitioners can non-threateningly inquire about a patient's sleep patterns.

## Change in Eating Patterns

Like sleep, eating is another sensitive biological indication of mental well-being. While both sleep and eating may be effected by physical illness per se, they are often also an indication of how well a person is coping. Problems in eating can be seen in decreased and increased appetite with an accompanying loss or gain of weight. These symptoms can also be readily seen, and noted for further analysis, in the hospitalized patient.

## Subjective Distress

While more difficult for an observer to notice, an increase in subjective or inner distress may be an early sign of the development of significant mental problems. Common uncomfortable feelings states include anxiety, depression, suspiciousness, irritability, and even inappropriate happiness. While the health practitioner may see the outward manifestations of these inner feelings, sensitive listening and questioning may be helpful. One key in considering such symptoms is whether they continue beyond the time of any real external trauma or whether they are inappropriate to the current situation. For instance, while most people may have some nervousness about the process of getting blood drawn, outright refusal, extreme pain, and perservation of concern after completion are all worth noting.

## Causing Distress in Others

Occasionally, the beginnings of mental problems may not be apparent in the clues already mentioned. In fact, the person may have no inkling within that something is wrong. Rather, their behavior will change to the extent that they will cause distress in other people. They will act differently than usual and not be aware of their change. A usually cooperative person may stop being easygoing at home, may be difficult to position properly for x-rays, and forget to pay medical bills. This kind of reaction to stress is especially common in children and adolescents. Children often lack a good understanding that they are experiencing emotional distress, and will commonly act out their problems in a variety of ways. Adolescents developing problems in coping may withdraw, get themselves in dangerous situations, or turn to drugs.

## General Problems in Love and/or Work

Problems in these main areas of living can, of course, indicate already existing mental problems. However, newly developed problems or a particularly long period of stagnation or frustration that can be controlled by the individual, may relate more to preventive possibilities. If we specifically consider the aspect of reaching potential, personal discovery may be a useful concept. Very often, there may be possible new ways ot solve an old problem, new relationships to develop, and new ways to look at oneself.

There are, of course, other warning signs to look for. Trouble in thinking is one. Memory problems is another. Hopwever, the general principle to remember is that any continuing change in a person's subjective sense of well-being or outward behavior is worth noting in a mental health check-up. Whether they are true indications of a beginning mental disorder needs to await further analysis by mental health professionals.


## EXAMPLES

Several examples may illustrate these clues for the allied health and nursing professional.

### "A Different Kind of Pain"

Mrs. X began to cry during a routine drawing of blood for lab work at the office. She had been feeling tired and weak for a few weeks, but did not really hurt anywhere in her body. Seeing the tears, the technician wasn't sure what to do, but decided to ask, "Am I hurting you, dear?" "No," the patient said. "It's not that kind of pain." "Can you tell me what kind?" The patient poured out her feelings about a marriage that was becoming more and more unsatisfactory. At the end of the conversation, the health professional mentioned that she had heard about these couples' groups where people could talk about these types of problems.

### "A Mother Can Do Too Much"

The mother was about 18 years old, and brought her infant son for his first check-up to the well-baby clinic. The medical assistant thought that the baby sucked hard at his bottle, but ignored his mother. The baby also looked thin and seemed to stare at the wall. The assistant said that it's usually hard to raise your first baby. The mother seemed to relax. The assistant then asked if the baby was gaining any weight. The mother said no, that she had tried breast feeding, but that the baby wouldn't eat enough. As they talked, the assistant noted that the mother seemed over-attentive in a peculiar way. The mother was in constant contact with her baby, pulling his fingers from her mouth, pressing her fingers firmly on the baby's head, rubbing and making red marks, and jerking her son suddenly. The assistant told the pediatrician, who found that the baby wasn't thriving and wondered about the possible development of child abuse. Arrangements were then made for more frequent visits and discussions with the assistant, help at home, and becoming involved with other parents. Unfortunately, we often hear about such hitting in retrospect after the injury or killing of babies by their parents.

### "Brain Waves"

An electroencephalogram (EEG) technician was applying the wires and electrodes to the man's head. He apparently had been acting somewhat oddly in the last few months. His question, "Are you planting thoughts in my head?" alerted the technician that a serious mental disorder may be developing. While it is natural to have fear and ignorance of the EEG, this question goes beyond that. The technician calmly replied, "No," explained the procedure, but relayed the information to the neurologist.

## REFERRALS

Once health professionals incorporate the concept of a mental health check-up into their usual activities, various responses may be necessary. The important task for the professional who is not a specialist in mental health is to try to recognize potential problems, not necessarily to do anything major themselves. Of course, listening itself may be therapeutic, but if one suspects the development of a mental disorder or the lack of development of potential, referral may be necessary.

Referring can be made in several ways. Sensitivity to, and anticipation of, the patient's reaction to this process is the key. The health professional can either alert their immediate supervisors or mention resources if they know of such. The patient should not feel as if they are being called crazy or being rejected by the health professional. The referral should be offered as a possible way to relieve distress, as indicated in the first example. Sometimes referrals need to be made quickly, for instance in situations with suicidal or homicidal potential, but often the process can be done gradually to alleviate the fears of the patient.

A general understanding of the various mental health specialists is useful for any practitioner. Moreover, the basic local mental health institutions should be known.

## CONCLUSIONS

The mental health check-up is basically an attitude that can enhance the health care role of any health practitioner. While the caregiver should never ignore their primary task, being alert to early signs of emotional distress and/or the absence of psychological well-being can add significantly to their impact. As part of the health care system, all caregivers are in unique situations were patients will trust them, even though they may be strangers. That trust needs to be used with sensitivity and care. Advice and counsel from mental health professionals is usually available.

Of course, in any primary prevention effort, the civil rights of the individuals must be considered. Any mental health intervention, even listening carefully for unrecognized problems, needs to respect the privacy and autonomy of patients and their families. If such cautions are remembered, providing bits of mental health check-ups will be rewarding to patients and their allied health and nursing caregivers.

## REFERENCES

1. Moffic HS, Adams GL (Eds.): A Clinician's Manual on Mental Health Care: A Multidisciplinary Approach. Menlo Park, CA: Adison-Wesley, 1982.

2. National Institute of Mental Health: Preventive Intervention in Schizophrenia. Rockland, MD, 1982.

3. Caplan G: Principles of Primary Prevention. New York: Basic Books, 1964.

# Chapter 17

## DIFFICULTIES IN WORKING
## WITH MENTAL HEALTH PROBLEMS

SETH W. SILVERMAN, M.D.
H. STEVEN MOFFIC, M.D.

Most allied health and nursing professionals will have contact with patients who have mental health problems. The difficulties that are experienced by both parties are multiple and complex. One of the major goals of this chapter is to help make some of these contacts a more positive and therapeutic experience. This goal may be achieved through a better recognition of some of the factors causing problems in reacting to mental health problems.

## THE STIGMA OF MENTAL ILLNESS

A stigma against mental patients has existed for a long time (1). Over the history of mankind, various things indicate they were treated in unusual and inappropriate ways. The burning to death of witches, exorcism, and torture were all once touted as "treatments." While current treatment seems more humane and successful, the stigma persists. The public often hears only of the rare violent individual, such as Charles Manson, Charles Whitman, and more recently in regard to President Reagan, John Hinckley. These people may or may not be psychiatric patients. In the language on the street, worlds like nuts, weird, wacko, crazy, flipped–out, and lunatic are still used quite commonly, even by health professionals. The fears of the mentally distrubed, as well as the fears of becoming mentally disturbed, may haunt all health professionals to some degree.

While the attitude of health professionals toward mental patients may differ somewhat from the general public, the negative feelings surrounding mental patients may still effect them. Health professionals may at least consciously want to help mental patients. However, (un)conscious fears may still lurk below the surface. In addition, family and friends may not give positive support for such work. Specific training in mental health care could help, but is often provided on a limited basis.

## LACK OF TRAINING

Health professionals, unlike mental health professionals, do not spend a great deal of time learning the rigors of psychiatric diagnosis and treatment. Most students in the mental health profession study their field exclusively between two and ten years. Mental health professionals can then use the psychiatric interview as the mainstay of psychiatric diagnosis. A comprehensive history and formal mental status examination are part of this process.

The health professionals's formal training in mental health may include only a one semester introductory course in psychology. This limited training may lead to several problems in the interface with mental patients. First, it may be hard to recognize when a patient is having mental problems. Especially if the problems are not severe, the allied health or nursing professional may feel uncomfortable because such problems may seem like normal problems that anyone, especially themselves, may have. The health professional observing an anxious patient may say to himself, "I often feel anxious like that myself." This may be followed by the following dangerous statement, "I can do it, why can't they?" Those feelings and thoughts we do not like in ourselves, we usually don't like to see in others. The patients may then be wrongly labeled as malingerers and/or trouble makers. Health professionals may then experience a wide range of emotions that interfere with the patient being viewed as sick and in need of help. Anger towards the patient may even be experienced by the health care provider.

One might recognize how difficult it is to treat such patients by introspectively asking, "Why would someone get me so angry that I do not want to do what I'm here for and more importantly, what do they need me for?" Second, without proper training, health professionals can feel quite helpless in knowing how to respond. Especially if patients are having major symptoms of depression or psychosis, not knowing how to react can be quite frightening.

## THE PAST MAY DISTORT THE PRESENT

Mental health professionals have found that patients who stimulate strong emotional responses in themselves may receive treatment that is more in accord with the mental health professional's needs than that of the individual they are treating.

This is usually the result of our own experiences and prejudices. From these biases we develop guidelines and sometimes rules on how to (re)act in similar situations. In other words, when we are presented with situations that seem similar to something that we have experienced in the past, we tend to use whatever behavior that allowed for a positive outcome in the previous experience, in the present one. This principle has direct applications in interactions with patients with mental disorders. We may tend to categorize individuals from our previous experiences and not treat them as individuals. We do this because it is easier. It is easier to rely on previous experiences than to treat each situation as if it was unique. This may save time and effort in the short run. However, we do this at the expense of generalizing and not allowing individuals to be just that, individuals.

One example of how we develop guidelines and rules and how this may effect our present day functioning may have to do with how each of us handles issues of authority. One of the first authority figures we experienced was our parents. We learned when no meant no, when no meant maybe, and when no really meant yes, but ask me another way or do it, just don't tell me. We also learned how to appreciate praise and conversely, respond to criticism from our parents. At some point in time, these reactions become internalized in our minds and we develop patterns of behavior. Probably one of the reasons the first grader does or does not listen to his teacher is because of how he or she relates to his parents. The same teacher may be perceived by different pupils as harsh, aggressive, mean or loving, kind and understanding. Other classmates may consider the teacher to be arrogant, gentle, patient or short-tempered. Each student may experience the teacher in a different and unique fashion according to his or her own previous experiences.

The psychiatric literature calls this phenomena transference. Transference is the re-enactment of previous and important relationships in a current relationship. How can this make sense? Are all the pupil–teacher relationships unique? Is it each pupil's perception of the teacher that is different, or does the teacher actually exhibit different behaviors to each and every student? Does the teacher have the same transference phenomena to the students? The answers are not easily found. In all probability, the teacher does not respond to all the pupils in exactly the same manner. She may have pupils she perceives as pets and she may have pupils she responds to as difficult or trouble makers. This may be also because of her previous experiences and what she expects from students who look or remind her of other pupils she has had in the past. The students may even remind the teacher of younger brothers or sisters. The students, on the other hand, probably respond to the teacher in a manner very similar to how they responded to their patients or other authority figures. They also may be able to get the teacher to respond in a manner very similar to that of their parents.

Growing older leads to more exposure to people and situations. We develop a more vaired and extensive repertoire of behavior. For most people, the principal in high school was thought to be a very smart and important man. You thought he or she ran the school and knew all the answers. If you are fortunate enough to meet the same individual 15 years later, your impression might be different. You might not feel that he was all powerful and you might even become aware that there were certain things that you could teach him. However, if you were locked in your own patterns of behavior and only could see him through the eyes of the high school student, you might not be able to understand how much you, and possibly he, had changed. So, in this case, the old pattern of reacting to him might interfere with your learning and seeing the situation as it really is.

All this is well and good, but what does this have to do with patients with emotional problems? If we continue with the example of reacting to authority, we can note that any health professional and patient interaction involves authority. From the patient's point of view, the allied health of nursing professional may represent past experiences with other authority figures. The patient may expect the caregiver to act in certain ways not based on how the caregiver really functions. In a simplified way, if the patient's mother was extremely nurturing, the patient may expect the caregiver to do everything. The patient may even perceive the caregiver as acting like that, when the caregiver is really acting in a different manner. These kinds of distortions can pose several problems for the caregiver. It can cause problems in communication. While it may be flattering to be idealized even if one does not deserve to be, such distortions can also cause the health professional to be inappropriately disliked. Patients get angry at caregivers because of inappropriate demands secondary to previous experiences and expectations. The expectations may not even be conscious to the patient and hence may not even be verbalized. Disillusionment may be felt by the patient as a general disregard on unsympathetic attitude on the part of the health care provider towards the patient. Generally, caregivers will have to handle being treated as if they were someone else.

If we turn to the professional's perception of the patient, this too can be subject to distortion. The caregiver may have a preconceived notion of what an authority figure (in this case health care professional) should be. This was probably formed by experiences with previous authority figures (like the principal). A rigid stance will result if caregivers do not modify their authoritarian role according to the situation. Patients will receive suboptimum care possibly experiencing rejection, anger and uncertainty. Also, certain patients may remind the caregiver of important people in the caregiver's life and interfere with a realistic assessment of the situation. The technical term for this is countertransference.

It is useful for the allied health and nursing professional to try to recognize when the past may be distorting current interactions. Rigid and rapid responses are often not helpful. Often, asking the opinions of other caregivers in these matters is useful. Each individual is a unique constellation of experiences, expectations, and emotions that will allow him or her to react to the obvious trauma of illness in a unique fashion. Patients (and caregivers) may react in other than their usual or preferred ways. Distortions will inevitably occur to some degree, but how we observe and use them is the key to satisfactory and satisfying work.

## PROBLEM PATIENTS

Patients who have certain kinds of behavior often are particularly likely to precititate strong emotional reactions in health professionals (2, 3). In fact, if the caregiver does not feel at least some unease with these patients, his own reaction should be questioned. This may be a symptom of the health care provider being overworked and not able to process new information. Conversely, a patient's emotional problems may be so frightening to the professional that he or she may deny their very existence. In the following section, we will attempt to categorize five types of such patients.

## Psychotic Patients

Psychotic patients are those patients who have impaired reality testing, or, in other words, seem to lose touch with reality. Psychosis may become evident to the health care provider by inappropriate and bizarre behavior on the part of the patient. This may be as obvious as the patient screaming and yelling at the top of his or her lungs that someone was out to get him and the only way he can protect himself is by hiding under the blankets. A more subtle psychotic state is the one that a primary care nurse may become aware of after many hours of intensive contact. An example is the individual who will only eat with the doors closed, so no one will watch or get him. Because disruptions in the perceptions of reality are so threatening to our own psyche, we tend to think of patients with these types of disturbances as incurable and inaccessible psychologically. Most patients with psychotic disorders do respond to some sort of verbal stimulation. Although the logic in which they respond to certain stimuli may not alsways be obvious to the provider, it does make sense to the patient on some level. The health care provider is advised to speak consistently and clearly. An attempt to understand what the precipitation for the psychosis is and what the patient feels may help alleviate some of his or her symptoms. Many secretive alcoholics are found out this way. A typical vignette is a male, middle-aged high level executive who comes into the hospital for the workup of a peptic ulcer. On the third day of hospitalization, he is noted by the nursing staff to become increasingly aware of his environment, hostile and maybe even paranoid. Later on in the evening, when the lights are turned out, he complains of green men and monsters crawling up his skin and the only way he can figure out to protect himself is by hiding himself in the bathroom with his pillow over his head. The immediate reaction of health professionals to this type of behavior may be one of repulsion or anger. However, if the change in behavior and the association to alcohol withdrawal is noted, the patient can be treated more appropriately and chance of immediate recovery is good.

## Dependent Patients

Another type of individual that can often be anxiety provoking and possibly anger producing for the health professional is that of individuals who manifest intense dependency needs. The behavior may be very subtle and range from a patient asking the nurse to get his slippers when he is able to do it himself, to the individual who gets angry at his doctor and refuses to eat. A form of dependent behavior can be found in an individual with passive aggressive personality traits. These individuals appear to be very passive as a way of provoking hostility and anger on the part of the health care provider. Patients may do this because they feel it is the only certain way not to be abandoned. This can be extremely vexing and is best seen in the example of an individual who for some reason is scared to take care of himself or herself because of the possible consequences. Another subtype of individuals who manifest dependent behavior are those who are very secretive. It is not unusual for a patient to become closely allied with one member of the health care team. At some point in time, the individual may appear to be disturbed and when asked about this state, say "I'd like to tell you something but you have to promise not to tell anybody." In an attempt to gain their trust and be helpful, the health care provider may indeed promise not to relay the information regardless of the content or importance. There is an inherent danger in this stance, in that by promising not to tell another individual of certain information this paralyzes the health care provider and may interfere with the information being used most appropriately. A more appropriate response when asked by an individual for total confidence is "I understand that the material you wish to tell me is very sensitive and I'll use it as best I can to help you." Besides these stressful behaviors, dependent patients often stir up our own feelings about not wanting to be vulnerable and mortal. Paradoxically, this may be some of the reasons we become health care professionals in the first place.

## Narcissistic Patients

Another type of difficult patient is the so-called "entitled" patient. These patients are very egotistical and narcissistic, which is evidenced by demanding and abusive behavior. The range of complaints vary from food being too hot or too cold, to the fact that their caregivers are never on time. These patients genuinely feel that the world should be their oyster. The more the health care provider goes out of his or her way to meet the unnecessary and extreme demands, the more the demands escalate. It is impossible to satisfy the inordinate and extreme demands of this type of individual. As a reaction to this, providers may not feel the need to respond to any demands. These patients are more appropriately responded to with specific limits, as well as clear and concise explanations as to why or why not certain things are being done for the patients.

## Chronic Complainers

Another type of patient that is frequently encountered is the so-called "help rejecting" patient. These patients ask for help in a variety of ways. When some sort of support or aid is offered, it is immediately rejected. Sometimes the rejection on the part of the patient is not immediately recognized, and the caregiver may rationalize this by saying that the patient didn't really understand. When these episodes repeat, the health care provider may feel inadequate and uncaring. Awareness of this subtle rejection on the part of the patient is foremost. Frequently, pointing out the paradoxical behavior to the patient may help both the patient and health provider deal with the patient's problems more effectively.

## Life-Threatening Patients

The patient who verbalizes suicidal or homicidal ideation can be extremely difficult. Both types of threats challenge our desire to save lives and help others. Suicidal potential is often not easy to assess, especially if the patient is reluctant to share the information with everybody. Generally, suicidal ideation should not be dismissed as being a game; rather the information should be handled sensitively and relayed to the appropriate supervisory personnel. Homicidal potential may feel like a danger to the caregiver's own life. It also may produce confidentiality dilemmas in knowing who and how to inform. Caution, calmness and careful assessment are all helpful responses. Again, dissemination of information to appropriate providers is appropriate and necessary.

## Case Examples

These five categories of patients are not inclusive and are only guidelines as to what type of behaviors patients manifest that may elicit strong emotional responses in allied health and nursing professionals. Generally responding to patients empathically, clearly and concisely will alay a lot of anxiety and fear on the part of the patient and caregivers. Explanations as to why certain procedures and tests are being ordered, as well as a genuine concern and interest in the welfare of the patient will help divert some of the more pathological energies on the part of the patient into more constructive avenues. Rarely do patients present with only one specific type of behavior and may indeed draw on behaviors from two or three of these categories at one time. It is important for the health care professional to be aware of what emotions he or she is experiencing and what are precipitating these feelings. Following are four vignettes that occurred in a hospital setting that may serve to illustrate these points.

### "Crazy or Not"

A sixty-four-year-old white female patient had been brought in by the police the night before because she was found walking the streets in her nightgown and could not answer them coherently. She had no identification, but was well groomed and did not appear to have any major problems. The patient was admitted. Because of some G.I. complaints a flat plate x-ray of the abdomen was ordered the next day. When the orderlies came the next morning, she was sleeping. They had heard from the morning supervisor that the patient was "psycho." After awakening, the patient refused to get onto the stretcher, which resulted in her sedation and involuntary transportation to x-ray. She fell off the stretcher in x-ray and broke her hip. After an operation and days of what was perceived by the staff to be extreme agitation, the patient finally became coherent. She asked the nurse where she was and how she got there. She was immediately able to contact her family. As the story unfolded, the patient revealed that the day of admission she had inadvertently taken too many sleeping pills and she wandered off. She appeared intoxicated and psychotic because of the accidental overmedication. When awakened by the orderlies she was understandably frightened and asked for clarification. The orderlies who had just finished restraining a patient on the psychiatry unit were "sure the best thing to do was to restrain the patient." In this case the police, medical personnel and radiology staff's expectations about a crazy elderly woman led to a disastrous outcome that in all probability could have been avoided by multiple interventions.

At the risk of playing Monday morning quarterback, what could have been done differently? The police might have asked the neighbors if they knew who the patient was and where she lived. The medical staff could have alerted nursing that the patient might have an organic brain syndrome and needed increased support, explanation and possibly primary care nursing. The orderlies might have tried to explain the procedure to the patient. When the orderlies met some resistance, they might have contacted the supervisor who then might have contacted the medical staff and delayed the procedure until the patient became more alert. The individuals concerned seemed to view the patient as a crazy, senile hopeless individual. If they had perceived her an an individual who became acutely ill and would recover, there might have been some effort on their part to modify their behavior and reaction more specifically to the patient, as opposed to reacting old memory tapes about previous experiences with perceived similar patients.

### "Anesthesia or Death"

Another vignette centers around a middle age female who comes into the hospital for an elective operation. On the night before the operation, she volunteers to the nurse on the 3–11 shift that she hopes she never recovers from the surgery. The patient breaks into tears and confesses an extramarital affair and states that she feels responsible for her husband leaving and the general disorder of her family. She states she "went shopping for a surgeon to do a hysterectomy on me," and hopes that she does not recover from the anesthesia. The nurse was obviously concerned and confused, and felt helpless. She was uncertain as to what to do with the information. Surgery was scheduled for the first think in the morning and she was not certain that the attending physician was aware of the previously stated information.

In this case, the most appropriate action on the part of the nurse would be to relay to the attending physician possible suicidal ideation on the part of the patient, and it then becomes the physician's responsibility as to how he or she chooses to handle such information.

### "The Patient Who Hurt Himself"

This vignette occurs in an intensive care unit. A reasonably healthy middle aged white male suffers his first heart attack and awakens after a two-day stormy course in the intensive care unit. The patient is aphasic and finds it difficult to communicate with his loved ones and caretakers. During the next 12 hours the nurse notes many malfunctions in his resuscitator. One instance she thinks she observes the patient actively reset some of the measurements, causing it to malfunction and sound the buzzer. She goes home and has difficulty sleeping that night and finally comes to the realization that somehow the patient is actively sabotaging his progress. She feels guilty and responsible and doesn't know what to do with the information.

In this case again, transmission of the information to appropriate supervisor and personnel would be the most appropriate action.

### "Health Professionals Are Human Too"

The next case involves the relatively common occurrence of a severely ill patient being resusitated in the emergency room. The physician was new to the hsopital and therefore unfamiliar with the emergency room and the personnel. Resusitation measures were instituted. However, the patient had fresh track marks in his antecubital fossa which were noticed by the nurse. The physician asked for input from the Code team. A nurse with whom he had previously quarreled snapped at him by stating, "Don't you think it's about time you checked for track marks?" The physician defensively stated that he already decided that was not the case. It was clear to the personnel involved that the physician was extremely threatened and did not appear to be responding in the most appropriate manner. The patient wasn't improving, and the physician complained that the other staff wasn't helping enough. Finally, after some delay, the patient was given appropriate therapeutic measures and began spontaneous respirations.

In this case, the physician could be categorized as "help rejecting." Although health caregivers are traditionally not labelled with patient behavior, the physician was clearly dependent and needy and allowed his own personal psychopathology (defensiveness) to interfere with appropriate treatment. What might have allowed for an optimum outcome would have been the recognition on the part of the physician that he is not omnipotent. The nurse in this case attempted to usurp the physician's authority and could have volunteered the information in a less confrontive and more informative manner.

## CONCLUSIONS

Working with mental health problems poses many problems. Since most allied health and nursing professionals will not have extensive formal training in this area, some guidelines may be helpful. First, be careful about stigmatizing patients who seem to be crazy or unusual. They may not be, and we may be distorting their behaviors. Moreover, even if they do have a severe mental illness. they invariably can be helped. Second, watch for particular kinds of problem patients. Patients who are psychotic, very dependent, overly narcissistic, help rejecting, and dangerous can tax the best of us. Using suggested treatment techniques and asking for  help can make working with mental problems more rewarding for everyone concerned.

## REFERENCES

1. Zilboorg G: A History of Medical Psychology. New York: WW Norton, 1941.

2. Main T: Psychiatric Defenses Against Close Encounter with Patients. Canadian Psychiatric Association Journal, 22:457–466, 1977.

3. Groves J: Taking Care of the Hateful Patient. New England Journal of Medicine, 298:883–887, 1978.

# Chapter 18

THE MENTAL HEALTH OF THE ALLIED HEALTH
AND NURSING PROFESSIONAL

SETH W. SILVERMAN, M.D.
H. STEVEN MOFFIC, M.D.

It is inevitable and expected that any health professional should experience some distress as the function of his or her primary employment. It is difficult to imagine how an individual exposed in some way to physical and mental illness on a day-to-day basis should not experience occasional feelings of inadequacy, dependency, and helplessness. Even the technician performing an isolated, repetitive mechanical task will in some way be aware of the importance to the anonymous patient. Indeed, if this were not the case, one might question whether a given individual is performing sensitively and empathically. It is the purpose of this chapter to help the individual first identify whether he or she is performing optimally. In addition, it is possible that the allied health and nursing professional may be able to identify those factors in their environment that are precipitating the emotional stress and decide what the most appropriate course of action should be. Attention to these issues will help the individual professional to reap the many possible rewards of the health field.

## JOB STRESS

Allied health and nursing professionals may, of course, be subject to the usual causes of mental health problems in anyone. However, there may be some aspects of being an allied health or nursing professional that are particularly stressful. Although more research needs to be done, there are indications of a high degree of job dissatisfaction in these fields (1).

Several factors have been identified as important contributors to any kind of job satisfaction (2). Necessary ingredients seem to be the opportunity for autonomy, upward mobility, promotions, and self-esteem. All these ingredients may be in particularly short supply in the allied health and nursing fields. Specifically, there are obvious limitations for autonomy in a physician led system. While many health professionals may feel comfortable in this kind of hierarchy, others may feel that they may not have enough authority and responsibility. More problematic and probably more pervasive are thoughts of having too much responsibility with too little autonomy and/or authority. Rightly or wrongly, cries of "we do all the work and they (the doctors) get all the credit" are not uncommon.

Institutions that train medical personnel, including physicians in residency training and medical students, as well as allied health and nursing professionals, are particularly susceptible to these job related stresses. Most medical students and residents obtain the majority of the clinical experiences in a sort of on-the-job training program. Medical students enter the clinical years with a wealth of book knowledge and intellectual curiosity. However, when it comes to actual clinical experience these highly trained, educated, and motivated individuals tend to resemble a "Bull in a China Shop" as opposed to promising young physicians. The majority of allied health and nursing professionals have more extensive clinical experiences as well as more practical ways of solving clinical problems than students of medicine. The threatened physician may become arrogant, hostile, abusive, or any one of a multitude of defense mechanisms to decrease their own feelings of inadequacy and/or inferiority. Allied health and nursing professionals may react similarly or attempt to intimidate or exaggerate their expertise because they finally have a chance to "get even." It is easy to see how any of these possible scenarios would result in increased job stress for both parties. Unfortunately, it is all too uncommon for individuals from differing fields with differing degrees of expertise and experience to work on a team together for the benefit of both patient and staff. Power struggles and pecking orders may interfere and at times dominate care for patients. In addition, medical personnel may at times forget that they are first and foremost human beings (just like other people) who have been fortunate enough to be in a profession entrusted with someone else's well being. Taking care of patients should be thought of as a privilege, not a right that comes with a certain title or degree.

Other sources of frustration may be limited opportunities for upward mobility and increased financial rewards. Here the cry may be "I could do more if they would only let me." Being from a minority group may make such limitations even more important.

In a relatively new field like allied health, other problems are common. Standards are rapidly evolving and changing. What was acceptable and standard practice yesterday may not be so today. This may leave individual workers insecure. Self–esteem may be shaken when one is not sure how well the job is being done. This may be due to lack of clearly defined job description and performance evaluation to unclear or unrealistic expectations on the part of the health care providers. Allied health and nursing professionals may appropriately feel ignored or unimportant when their input into these matters is not utilized.

## RECOGNITION OF PERSONAL PROBLEMS

The most important initial step in evaluating abnormal amounts of stress in the allied health and nursing professional is for the individual to acknowledge that he or she is not performing adequately. However, due to the complexity of human feelings and interactions, this assessment or acknowledgement is often easier said than done. Patients, supervisors and individuals themselves may consciously be aware that a problem exists but may not be able to pinpoint the source. Fears of reprisal and scapegoating may also serve to temporarily camouflage a suboptimally performing worker.

Inevitably, indications of distress surface in a variety of different contexts. For instance, the allied health care professional may not be sleeping well at night and/or having frequent nightmares. Another common occurrence is an increased amount of perceived stress, especially within intimate relationships. There may be an increased usage of alcohol, medicine, and illicit drugs. Physical illness may occur and seemingly minor ailments may take a new, greater importance in the life of a stressed health care professional. Frequent trips to physicians, without any apparent resolution of symptoms may be another stress warning sign. Changes in level of physical exercise, and more specifically sexual activity, may serve as another barometer. Stressed individuals may also avoid contacts with friends and extended family and attempt to limit daily activities to minimize contact with the outside world. At work, individuals may notice increased tardiness, anticipating breaks with greater fervor, absenteeism, and longing for the end of the day. They may begin to avoid their peers and not participate in various professional activities. Interest in continuing education as well as enthusiasm to teach newer colleagues may also wane. Some individuals may just note that they are generally more easily provoked and less friendly. On rare occasions, the individual may even feel too good, too confident, or too assured. This may be due to denying the existence of painful, lonely feelings that plague us all to certain degrees.

The next step in attempting to solve these types of difficulties after admitting their existence is to seek help. This indeed may be the most difficult task as many people may choose to go into this specific profession because of their needs to help other people. They may incorrectly think that if they have some sort of difficulty themselves, they can no longer be of service to others. A common saying among psychotherapists with regard to their own personal psychopathology is "The best of us get treatment and the worst of us use our patients." It is often frightening for health care professionals to experience some of the stresses, vulnerabilities, and difficulties that they incorrectly assumed they are immune to. In reality, these sensitivities and vulnerabilities when allowed to come into conscious awareness may provide for a learning experience that allows the individual to become more effective professionally and personally. The syndrome of "burn-out" is due to some inability to become aware of these stresses as they occur and to understand them. The individual becomes overwhelmed, can no longer sort out what factors are responsible for which feelings and lumps the entire syndrome together as "burn-out." Individuals who change jobs and locations find that they suffer burn-out in the new environment because the same unresolved stresses eventually reappear.

Unfortunately, there are often no precise or absolute indications of knowing when to get mental health care. Nevertheless, it is better to go early than late. At the very least, self-knowledge can be improved and at the very best resolution of symptoms with increased personal and professional satisfaction will ensue.

## HOW TO GET HELP

What can the health care professional do once she or he becomes aware of the fact that they are not performing their job with the same enthusiasm or level of performance? Staff meetings and staff interactions can be a unique source of support. Sharing the difficulties with staff regarding problem patients allows for brain storming with possible solutions of a more diversified, effective, and unified treatment approach. If there are difficulties with supervisors and peers, they should be handled initially at the level of the unsatisfactory interaction. Friends and family may serve as a source of support and understanding. However, at times this burden may become unfair and individuals should be aware of the fact that they may be scapegoating noninvolved people.

It is difficult to underestimate the importance of the general well–being of the health care professional. Regular physical "tune-ups," including exercise, good diet, and adequate amounts of sleep, do wonders for mental health. Psychologically, too often we become involved in repetitive patterns that do not allow for us to seek new solutions for old problems. Outside interests, whether they be hobbies or continuing education, tend to constructively stimulate our own psyches. With added emotional reserve, the probability of unique solutions for chronic or acute problems improve.

At some point in time, it may become obvious to the individual, peers, supervisors or family members that particular stresses are not being adequately resolved by the previously discussed methods. In this case, mental health care professionals should be sought out. It is a curious paradoxical occurrence that people who spend a great majority of their time taking care of other individuals should be so resistant to acknowledging their own difficulties and seeking appropriate care.

There are varied approaches to treating emotional illness or mental disturbances. Whether the individual finds group therapy, couples therapy, individual therapy, family therapy, and/or medication to be most beneficial will depend upon his or her unique circumstances. Usually that decision can be made with the advice of the mental health professional.

Some individuals fear that seeking professional attention inevitably implies a terminal emotional illness that can only be supported and will result in chronic dependence upon the mental health provider. This bias may contribute to the stigma attached to psychiatry found in the general population. Individuals who function at a reasonable level of competence and find that for some reason they can no longer do so, can expect some degree of symptom relief and restitution of function by seeking professional care.

## CONCLUSIONS

There are numerous rewards to be found in the work of allied health and nursing professionals. These range from basic financial remuneration to the privilege of being involved in caring for those needing help. Allied health professionals are also part of the excitement produced by the development of a new field. All these rewards, however, may be jeopardized if health professionals ignore their own mental well-being and that of their patients.

Work in the allied health and nursing fields is not easy. So, in addition to the life's usual problems, professionals in these areas are often subject to extra stress. Several sources of help are available. Support from peers, supervisors, and family can often be useful. If not, overcoming fears of asking for professional psychiatric care can later prove to be invaluable. Attention to the mental well-being of the health professional will usually correlate with increased professional and personal satisfaction and success.

## REFERENCES

1. Broski DC, Cook S: The Job Satisfaction of Allied Health Professionals. J Allied Health, 7:281, 1978.

2. Dunnette M (Ed.): Handbook of Industrial Psychology and Organizational Behavior. Chicago: Rand McNally, 1976.

# ADDITIONAL ANNOTATED REFERENCES


1. Abbott AA: Professional Choices—Values at Work. Silver Spring, MD: National Association of Social Workers, Inc., 1988. Discusses how our professional and personal values influences our work.

2. American Psychiatric Association: Diagnostic and Statistical Manual of Mental Disorders, Third Edition, Revised (DSM-III-R). Washington, D.C.: American Psychiatric Press, 1987. The most recent update on the major diagnostic classification scheme for psychiatric problems in the United States.

3. Avraham R: Substance Abuse—Prevention and Treatment. New York: Chelsea House, 1988. This easily read book covers the essentials of what has been called a mental health "epidemic."

4. Berger DM: Clinical Empathy. New Jersey: Jason Aronson, 1987. An in-depth discussion of the crucial ingredient for understanding our patient's problems.

5. Bowder CL, Burstein AG (Eds): Psychosocial Aspects of Health Care. Baltimore: Williams and Wilkins, 1983. Covers the omnipresent psychological component of any health problem.

6. Comas-Diaz L, Griffith, EEH (Eds): Clinical Guidelines in Cross-Cultural Mental Health. New York: John Wiley & Sons, 1988. The most practical reference for how to incorporate the cultural variable in our pluralistic patient population.

7. Haubrich DI, McLead DW: Psychosocial Dimensions of HIV and AIDS: A Selected Annotated Bibliography. Ottawa, Canada: Federal Center for AIDS (Bonaventure Bldg., 2nd Fl. 301 Elgin St., Ottawa, Canada, KIA OL2), 1988. Covers the multiple new references on the mental health aspects of our most significant new health problem.

8. Haugard JJ, Reppuci ND: The Sexual Abuse of Children. San Francisco: Jossey-Bass, 1988. Comprehensive coverage of an increasingly discussed, but still difficult to recognize, mental health problem.

9. Henao S, Grose NP (Eds): Principles of Family Systems in Family Medicine. New York: Brunner Mazel, 1985. Edited by both a psychiatrist and family practitioner, this book elaborates on what we now know concerning how health issues affect not only patients, but also their families.

10. Hyman SE, Arana GW: Handbook of Psychiatric Drug Therapy. Boston: Little, Brown, and Co., 1987. A pocket size, reasonably up-to-date reference for the use of medications for mental health problems.

11. Krueger DW (Ed): Rehabilitation Psychology. Rockville, M.D.: Aspen Publications, 1984. Covers the role of all mental health and health professionals in medical rehabilitation services.

12. Lion, JR, Adler WN, Webb WL (Eds): Modern Hospital Psychiatry. New York: Norton, 1988. Discusses the setting where multidisciplinary teamwork is so essential for mental health care.

13. Reiser SJ, Bursztaja, Appelbaum, PS, Gutheil TG: Divided Staffs, Divided Selves—A Case Approach to Mental Health Ethics. Cambridge: Cambridge U. Press, 1987. From sex to selling out, this casebook covers practical issues concerning the increasingly recognized ethical component of all mental health care.

14. Robin HS, Michelson JB (Eds): Illustrated Handbook of Drug Abuse. Chicago: Year Book, 1988. Showing the physical manifestations of substance abuse should be of particular help to nursing and allied health professionals.

15. Tardiff K: Concise Guide to Assessment and Management of Violent Patients. Washington, D.C.: American Psychiatric Press, 1989. Will help to preserve the physical well-being of all of us!

16. Vinogradov S, Yalom ID: Concise Guide to Group Psychotherapy. Washington, D.C.: American Psychiatric Press, 1989. Written for the clinician, this short volume offers practical advice on using groups.

# INDEX

## P

Paranoid disorders, 85–86
Personality assessment, 99–100
   minority patients, 109
   tests, 104–107
Personality disorders, 91–92
Prevalence of mental illness,
   235–236
Pseudodementia, 16
Psychiatrists, 231
Psychoanalysis, 125, 129
Psychoanalytic psychotherapy,
   130–131
   for mental health professionals,
     210
Psychologists, 97–98, 231–232
Psychosexual development, 35–36
Psychosexual disorders, 88–89
Psychosis, 120–122, 254–255
   antipsychotic medication, 122
   psychosocial intervention, 122
Psychotherapists, 128
   effective traits, 202

## R

Rapid tranqulization, 118, 121
Referrals, 67
   resistance to, 228–231
Reinforcers, 143–145, 150
Relaxation techniques, 147–148
Restraints, 117–118

## S

Schizophrenia, 7–9, 85–86
   loose associations, 78
   psychodynamics of, 41
Seclusion rooms, 118
Self-harm, 259
Sexual history, 75–76
Sleep patterns, 242–243
Slips of the tongue, 39
Social network, 217
Social workers, 232

Somatoform disorders, 87
Speech, 78–79
Stimulant medication, 177–179
Stigma, 228, 249–250, 266
Stress, 214–216
   for health professionals,
     261–263
Substance abuse, 11–13
Suicide, 113–116, 256
   depression and, 114
   management, 115–116
   organicity and, 115
   personality and, 115
   psychosis and, 114
   risk factors, 113
Superego, 36–37
Supervision, 208–209
Suspicious patients, 31–32
Sympathy, 127

## T

Tardive dyskinesia, 161–162
Teamwork (see Multidisciplinary
   teamwork)
Token economy, 150
Transference, 127
   problems in health care,
     251–253
Treatment refusal, 62

## V

Values, 58–59

## W

Warning signs, 242–244
   in children, 243